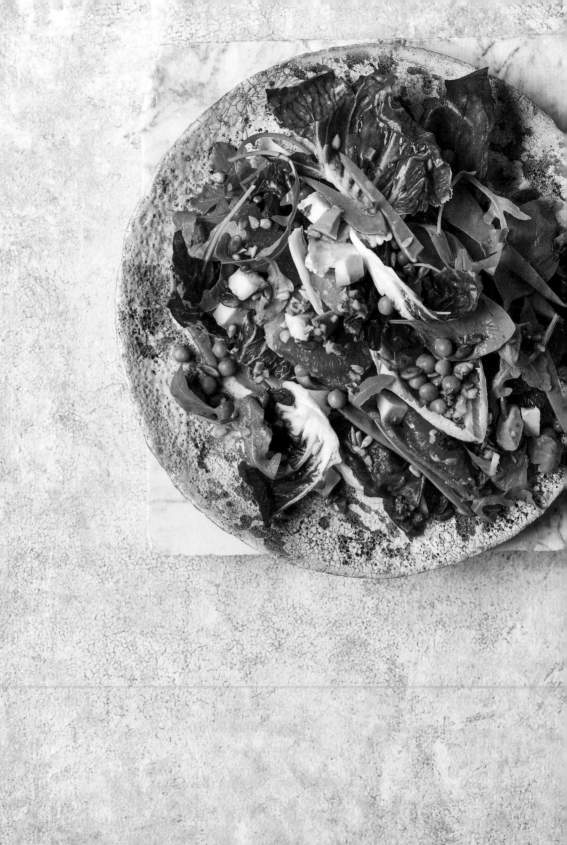

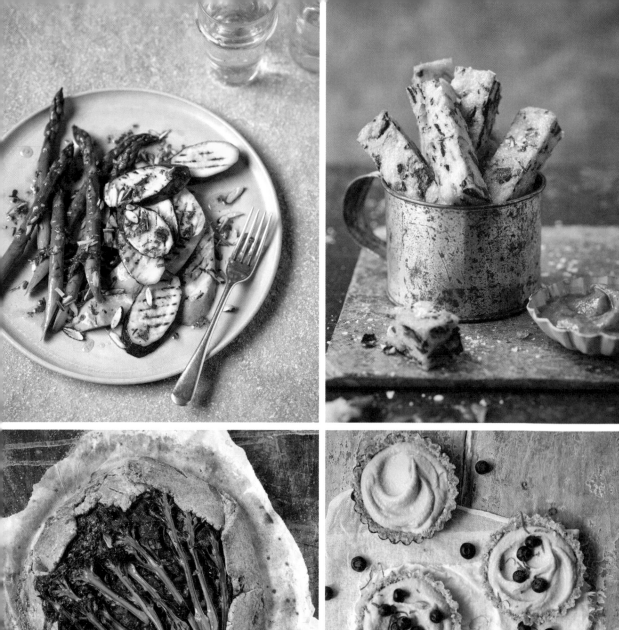
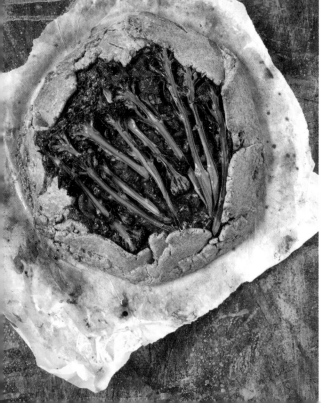
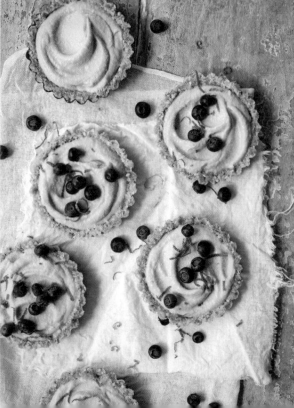

Eat More Greens

The most inventive recipes
to help you eat more greens

ZITA STEYN

Photography by Nassima Rothacker

quadrille

For my mom, whose dedication to the wellbeing of her loved ones has never wavered. Ever.

Recipe notes

When budget, availability and time allow, I recommend the following:

- organic meat, dairy products, gelatin and eggs from humanely treated animals that have been pastured and allowed to roam free
- good-quality stock, preferably homemade
- sustainable seafood from unpolluted waters
- raw (or unpasteurized) cider vinegar, dairy products, coconut oil and water, and honey
- extra-virgin olive oil and other good-quality cold-pressed oils
- organic or minimally sprayed fresh local and seasonal produce, preferably biodynamically grown
- organic unwaxed citrus fruits, especially if zesting
- organic and preservative-free ingredients, such as condiments, sausages, wine, coconut milk and dried fruit (sweetened with fruit juice, if at all)
- filtered water, especially when used for fermenting or preserving
- soaking (and even sprouting) grains, nuts, seeds and legumes before cooking and/or consuming

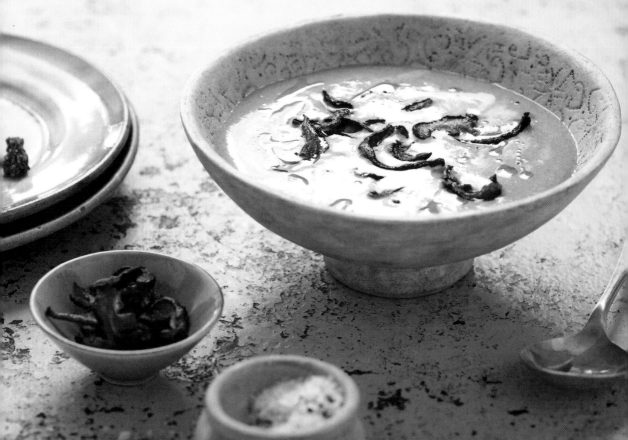

Contents

Introduction

My approach to food has been largely shaped by my upbringing in an active, unfussy, and lively household. My mother had always taken her responsibility of feeding us, her four boisterous children, extremely seriously, and although I was slightly embarrassed at the time, I still recall the feeling of awe every time I opened a lunch box she had prepared. When I was at primary school, my mom fell ill with chronic fatigue syndrome for several years, and only managed to claw her way out of the black hole by implementing a complete overhaul of her—and our!—lifestyle. It meant studying nutrition and holistic medicine in great depth, drastically reducing sugar and refined foods even more, and preparing meals that withstood the rigorous test of being whole, wholesome, and health-supportive. But amazingly the food still tasted fantastic!

This book was born out of the one question that almost all my clients and friends have asked me at some point: "How do I incorporate more green vegetables into my diet?" That was all the inspiration I needed to create this collection of honest, delicious, and interesting dishes based on a real need by real people.

Green vegetables, in particular the dark-green leafy kind, are the most nutrient-dense foods available to us. They contain an array of potent compounds that are very difficult to find anywhere else in the same concentration. Green vegetables are rich in dietary fiber, folic acid, beta-carotene, vitamin C, vitamin K, potassium, and magnesium, as well as containing a host of phytochemicals that can reduce inflammation and eliminate carcinogens. They contain a variety of carotenoids, flavonoids, and other powerful antioxidants that prohibit the oxidation of molecules in the body and are thought to prevent several degenerative diseases. Some green vegetables are also a major source of iron and calcium. In addition to these, sea vegetables (many of them a dark green-black), contain all of the 56 elements essential for human health in bioavailable form, together with important trace elements like selenium that are often lacking in land vegetables due to soil demineralization.

Over 2,000 years ago, Hippocrates said that all illness begins in the gut. And today many experts still believe there is a lot of truth in that. How can we expect to power our hard-working engines if we don't prioritize the fuel we put into them? Some of the recipes in this book may use a few more ingredients and seem a little more time-consuming than you are used to, but they are certainly not difficult to make and they are well worth the effort. Anyone can put something on a plate and call it supper, but only those who know how to combine flavors and use all the varied aromatics nature has to offer, will serve up a meal that is not only medicine for the body, but also food for the soul.

Zita

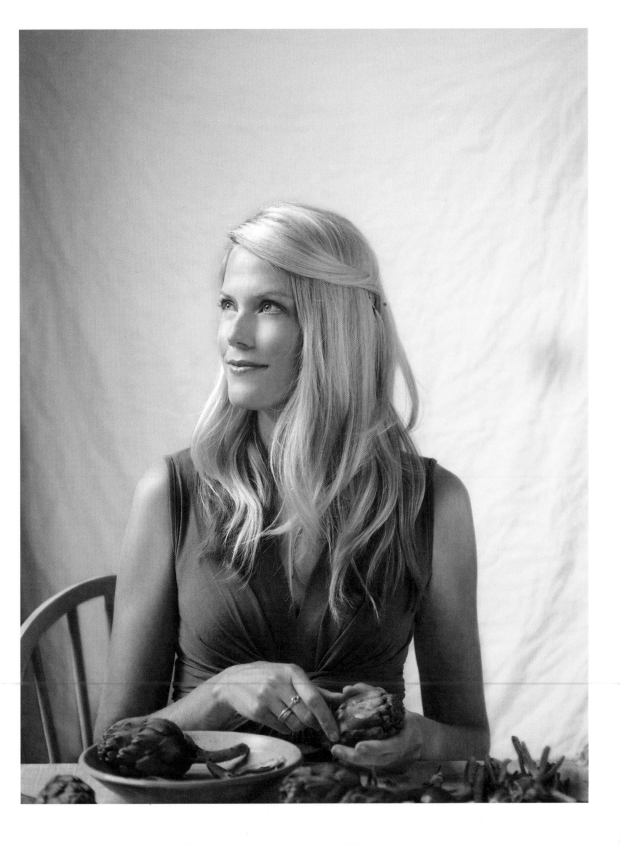

Green champions

It is wonderful to see how the tide is turning and that ever more people are becoming aware of the crucial role that good, nutritious food plays in a healthy life. Most of us now know that eating lots of vegetables, especially green ones, is vital. One question I often get asked, however, is how to incorporate these green vegetables on a daily basis. And so the idea for this book was born. In it you will find suggestions on how to use many different kinds of green vegetables, with a particular focus on leafy greens. Feel free to substitute and experiment—once you are familiar with these wonderful foods, you will no doubt find many more ways to enjoy them!

A word of advice: try not to get stuck on a few trusty friends. It is important to rotate between all the different vegetables, because each belongs to a different family that boasts a unique nutritional profile. Dark-green leafy vegetables are high in calcium and iron, and the bioavailability of the calcium is actually higher in kale and other dark-green leafy vegetables (like broccoli) than in dairy, but you need to eat a large variety of calcium-containing plant foods to ensure you are getting enough. Many vegetables also contain small amounts of toxins as a defense mechanism to protect the plant against predators. If consumed in excess these toxins could have a negative impact on your health, for example, the goitrogens in cruciferous vegetables could interfere with thyroid hormone function in susceptible individuals, and the oxalic acid in—among others—spinach, chard and beet greens may inhibit mineral absorption and lead to kidney stone formation in those prone. Rotating between them will therefore ensure you gain the maximum advantage of all the wonderful nutrients they have to offer, without building up harmful levels of any toxin.

Aquatic greens

These are greens that live and grow in or near water. If they are not yet a regular part of your diet, consider finding ways to include them often. Remember to source aquatic greens from clean waters.

SEAWEEDS

Green sea vegetables are extremely nutritious, as they offer one of the broadest ranges of minerals of any food, containing almost all the minerals found in the ocean, including iodine, copper, iron, zinc, potassium, phosphorus, and manganese. They contain a variety of unique phytonutrients, including the potent fucoidans, that appear to have antitumor, anticancer, and neuro-protective actions. Unlike some other categories of vegetables, sea vegetables do not appear to depend on carotenoids and flavonoids for their antioxidant benefits because they contain several other types, including alkaloid antioxidants. Sea vegetables are also an excellent source of vitamins A, C, thiamin, riboflavin, niacin, and B6.

WATERCRESS

Spidery watercress—well known to many as a garnish and almost always pushed to one side by diners—is not only one of the most nutrient-dense foods available to us, but its peppery leaves are also very exciting to eat and cook with. Although this plant is technically a member of the brassica family (see page 10) and botanically related to garden cress, arugula, and mustard, I have included it in this group, as it is considered an aquatic or semiaquatic perennial plant that is often found near slow-moving water. Among the oldest-known leafy greens consumed by humans, watercress contains significant amounts of iron, calcium, iodine, and folic acid, as well as vitamins A and C. It is great in salads and soups, tossed with pasta, on sandwiches, and paired with citrus or seafood, especially smoked fish. The best way to buy and store watercress is in lush bunches and in a small pitcher of water.

SAMPHIRE

A distinction is made between rock samphire, found on cliffs or in rocks and shingle on the Mediterranean coast, and marsh samphire (also known as sea beans, sea asparagus, or glasswort), a succulent that also grows near the sea, but prefers estuaries and wetlands rich in minerals and trace elements. Samphire is a good diuretic, believed to aid digestion, and is rich in vitamin C. Choose stalks that are bright green and firm, wash them well, and use as soon as possible. They only need a minute or two of steaming or stir-frying, but can be enjoyed raw too. Remember not to add any salt to the dish, as samphire is very salty.

SIMPLE WAYS TO EAT AQUATIC GREENS:

1. Combine *watercress* with other lettuces in a salad with sliced oranges and avocados, and serve with a simple vinaigrette.

2. Sprinkle a pinch of dried *kelp* flakes into soups or stews while cooking.

3. Make a side dish with quinoa, finely chopped herbs, and *watercress*, chopped tomatoes, and minced onions. Add lemon juice, olive oil, and salt.

4. Rinse *arame* and soak for 5 minutes, before adding to sautéing vegetables such as carrots, slow-cooked onions, winter squash, lotus root, and some shiitake mushrooms.

5. Sauté garlic and *samphire* for a minute, then add slivers of lightly steamed asparagus. Serve with a drizzle of olive oil.

6. Chop and simmer together a bunch of *watercress*, a couple of pears, garlic, onions, a potato or two, and some ginger in a pot with broth, then blend until smooth for a revitalizing soup.

7. Chopped, rehydrated *hijiki* and *arame* are delicious added to cooked rice, millet, or barley.

8. Make a *watercress* sauce for broiled fish by mixing finely chopped watercress, lemon juice, crème fraîche or thick plain yogurt, and sea salt.

9. Toast *nori* sheets in a hot pan and eat as a snack.

10. Finely chop *samphire* and add to a kedgeree a minute before serving.

Green brassica (or cruciferous) vegetables

Pungent, potent brassicas—all members of the mustard family—are the undisputed heavy-hitters in the vegetable world. Not only is almost every part (root, stalk, stem, leaf, bud, flower, sprout, and seed) of a plant used for food in this family, they are also rich in vitamins, minerals, and antioxidants, and contain very high levels of phytochemicals, the non-nutritive substances in plants that have been shown to fight carcinogens, inflammation, and liver toxicity, and generally support good health. Most brassicas improve taste-wise, and become less pungent and more digestible, with gentle cooking, such as steaming, or a brief sauté.

KALE, CURLY KALE, AND TUSCAN KALE

In addition to providing high levels of vitamins and flavonoids, superheroes kale & co. contain several natural components (called glucosinolates) that are converted into sulfur-containing phytochemicals (called isothiocyanates) in the digestive tract, and these in turn are thought to help prevent several types of cancer and, in some cases, even suppress the growth of cancerous tumors. Thanks to their broad nutritional profile, these vegetables are also believed to help fight cardiovascular disease, asthma, rheumatoid arthritis, and premature aging of the skin, and to promote the health of the urinary tract. Finally, all common kale cultivars provide plenty of carotenoids which, among others, are known for their ability to support eye health. Tuscan kale is called black cabbage cavola nero, dinosaur kale, or lacinato.

COLLARD GREENS

These spring cabbages are similar to kale in that the central leaves only form a very loose head, thus giving us silky, easy-to-prepare leaves without the crunch of round cabbages. Being loose, all the leaves are fully exposed to light, and so more strongly flavored, but are also particularly rich in vitamin C, folic acid, and dietary fiber. They are considered to be closer to wild cabbage than most other domesticated forms.

ARUGULA AND MUSTARD GREENS

Arugula is an annual herb that varies from mild in flavor and similar to baby spinach in appearance when young, to peppery, bitter and with elongated lobular leaves when mature. Mustard greens (also called Indian or Chinese mustard, and leaf mustard) are the greens of a subspecies of the mustard plant and also very peppery, although cooking does reduce this. Like most other dark leafy greens, arugula and mustard greens are a great source of vitamins A, B-complex, C, and K, as well as folates.

GREEN CABBAGES AND BRUSSELS SPROUTS

Common green (and red) cabbages, one of the oldest of the brassica vegetables, and the ancestors of broccoli and cauliflower, have thick leaves and round, tightly wrapped heads. Savoy cabbage has a milder flavor and thinner, more textured leaves. Brussels sprouts look like tiny cabbages, but are in fact buds that form all along tall stalks of the parent plant. Cabbages, like other brassicas, are high in sulfur and rich in phytonutrients antioxidants.

BROCCOLI

Broccoli (regular, tenderstem, and broccoli rabe or rapini) contains one of the most powerful phytochemicals — sulforaphane—which is formed when the vegetable is cut, chopped, and/or chewed. Bacteria in your intestines can also act on broccoli to produce sulforaphane. This phytochemical is so potent that scientists are interested in developing it as a potential treatment for cancer and autism. Unfortunately frozen broccoli lacks the ability to produce sulforaphane, but researchers are working on a solution, for example adding a small amount of radish powder to the frozen veg.

ASIAN BRASSICAS (BOK CHOY, CHINESE BROCCOLI, TATSOI, NAPA CABBAGE, AND MIZUNA)

These are similar in some ways to the more familiar European brassicas, but are faster growing, often more productive and have many and varied uses. Most parts are eaten, used in stir-fries, or steamed, but they can also be used as salad greens. Flavors vary from mild to peppery, but they are generally not as pungent or bitter as the other brassicas. Napa cabbage, also called Chinese or celery cabbage, has a more delicate texture and flavor than common cabbage.

ROOT BRASSICAS (KOHLRABI AND WASABI)

The name "kohlrabi" is an amalgamation of the German word for cabbage and the Swiss German word for turnip—and this is a good description of the taste you can expect. I love it raw, either finely chopped, grated, or as carpaccio, but it can also be sautéed, roasted, or added to stir-fries and stews. The greens are also delicious raw (when young and tender) or wilted.

Wasabi is commonly known as Japanese horseradish, although it is not from a species of horseradish, but rather a brassica. Although wasabi does have a strong, spicy taste, it is different from the taste of chile peppers, which get their heat from capsaicin that causes a "burning" sensation on the tongue. Wasabi releases chemical vapors that affect the nasal passage. The powerful smell and taste are derived from the high levels of isothiocyanate, the sulfur-containing phytochemical which is believed to combat cancer.

SIMPLE WAYS TO EAT GREEN BRASSICAS:

1. Serve sautéed or steamed *broccoli* or other brassicas with blank canvas foods, such as cooked legumes or rice, and lots of olive oil.

2. Any kind of fat can be used to subdue the flavor of an ingredient, as well as add richness and a wonderful mouth-feel to any dish. Try adding coconut cream to a *kale* and chicken curry, for example, or mixing some nuts and avocado into your dressed *mustard green* and *lettuce* salad.

3. Brassicas are delicious with a variety of chiles or cayenne pepper, and one of my favorite ways with *bok choy* is to sauté it with some salt, garlic, and chopped chiles in a little oil, then to toss it with cooked soba noodles. Serve this with virgin sesame oil and sesame seeds.

4. Adding creamy organic (preferably pastured and unpasteurized) dairy products, such as soft cheese, cream, or yogurt, to a *brassica* stir-fry or soup, or a dressing intended for a *arugula* salad, makes all the difference.

5. Bold flavors do well alongside salty ingredients, such as olives, hard cheeses, anchovies, smoked or cured meats, and fish, capers, and shoyu. Try grating some Parmesan over an oven-roasted tray of *Brussels sprouts*.

6. I love the taste of *cabbage* with fruit —raw cabbage with fresh fruit such as an apple and shaven cabbage salad, or sautéed cabbage with dried fruits such as raisins or currants.

7. Try shredding some *spring greens* and frying in a little oil before tossing in a tangy lemon and honey vinaigrette. Adding something sweet to pungent foods often helps balance the flavor.

The beet family

Spinach, chard, and all the beet cultivars belong to the Amaranth (or Amaranthaceae) family, which is mostly native to tropical America and Africa. This flowering plant family is dominated by herbs but also includes vines, shrubs, and trees. Leaves are mostly simple and entire, and flowers regular, cyclic, and tiny.

SPINACH

Believed to have originated in Persia, spinach spread across Europe by the 12th century and was desirable for its healthful properties even in those days. Generally you will find two or three different types of spinach: Savoy, with dark-green wrinkled leaves, semi-savoy, and a flat-leaf type with smooth leaves. Fresh leaves are a rich source of antioxidants, vitamins A and C, flavonoids, and carotenoids, which together help protect against free radicals. This green leafy vegetable and its family members also contain good amounts of many B-complex vitamins and vitamin K, as well as being a good source of potassium, manganese, magnesium, copper, zinc, and iron. One thing to note with this group of vegetables is the concentration of oxalic acid (especially in more mature plants), which is present but much lower in many other vegetables and plant-based foods, but high enough in this family to interfere with the absorption of minerals such as calcium and iron. To avoid this, rotate your greens, mix high-oxalate greens with lower-oxalate greens, cook the greens and discard the cooking water, or ferment them. On top of that, iron from plant sources (called non-heme iron) as compared to animal sources (heme iron) is quite difficult for your body to absorb, so add some vitamin C-rich foods such as peppers and citrus, or some heme-iron foods to your meal to increase the iron absorption, and avoid foods that may inhibit iron absorption, such as calcium-rich foods, caffeine, cocoa, phytate-rich foods (such as soy, some nuts and seeds, and some legumes), and eggs.

SWISS OR RAINBOW CHARD

Chard (also known as Swiss chard, leaf beet, silver beet, spinach beet, seakale beet, crab beet, mangold, and even just spinach in some countries) is a leafy green vegetable with large leaves that taste a little like spinach, but are slightly sweeter. Younger leaves can be eaten raw in salads, but the fleshy stalks and tougher leaves of more mature plants are usually cooked. Like spinach, chard is full of phytonutrients, vitamins, and minerals, and should be briefly boiled or sautéed to retain as many of these as possible. The leaf can be green or reddish and the stalks also vary in color—usually white, yellow, or red (which is what "rainbow chard" refers to).

SIMPLE WAYS TO EAT THE BEET FAMILY:

1. When making gnocchi from scratch, add some pureed *spinach* and grated nutmeg to the dough.

2. Finely shred *beet greens* and add to a beet and chickpea curry a few minutes before serving.

3. Add a handful of *spinach* leaves and some sautéed onion to two beaten eggs for an easy breakfast scramble.

4. Juice younger *beet greens* together with lower oxalate lettuces and add a lemon to increase iron absorption.

5. Make a version of the Punjabi potato and *spinach* dish, aloo-palak, by sautéing a bay leaf, pinch of ground cloves, and some ground cinnamon and turmeric until fragrant, then adding chopped onions, garlic paste, and grated ginger, and cooking this with chopped tomatoes until soft. Stir in finely chopped, cooked spinach and cubed cooked potatoes, and season to taste.

6. Cook the stems and leaves of *rainbow chard* until tender, then finely shred and stir into lightly steamed carrots and peas with a little bit of salted butter.

7. Top crispy rye toast with sautéed *beet greens*, soft goat cheese, fresh figs, and a drizzle of aged balsamic vinegar.

8. Use briefly blanched large-leaf *spinach* or *chard* leaves to make packages filled with cooked lentils, onion, chopped fresh herbs, grated ginger, and spices, such as paprika and allspice.

9. *Swiss chard*, caramelized onions, and goat cheese are great together in a tart or quiche.

The daisy family

The Asteraceae or Compositae *(commonly known as the aster, daisy, or sunflower family) are a large family of flowering plants with over 23,600 species and 13 subfamilies. Many members have composite flowers in the form of flower heads, like the star form of its most prominent member, the aster. This family provides us with valuable products such as cooking oils, lettuces, sunflower seeds, artichokes, sweetening agents, coffee substitutes, and herbal teas and medicines.*

LETTUCES, LEAVES, AND BITTER GREENS

Many edible lettuces and leaves fall in the daisy family, including curly endive (or frisée), romaine, cos, chicory or Belgian endive, escarole, radicchio, oak leaf, dandelion, butter (Bibb and Boston) lettuce, iceberg, and loose-leaf lettuce. The leaves all boast different shapes, sizes, colors, textures, and tastes. Generally the darker green the leaf, the more nutritious, but they are all a wonderful addition to your diet, being rich in chlorophyll, antioxidants, vitamins, and minerals (specifically potassium, calcium, phosphorous, iron, and magnesium), and very low in oxalic acid.

Lettuces range in bitterness from mild (such as butter lettuce) to severe (like dandelion or chicory), but don't be put off by it. Like many other green vegetables already discussed, the bitterness in edible leaves triggers a chemical reaction in our bodies that has numerous health benefits, such as helping to absorb nutrients by stimulating the production of gastric acid, enzyme production, and bile flow. Bitter foods also help balance taste buds, control food cravings, and help sweep waste through the digestive tract with the help of fiber and sulfur-based compounds which support the natural detoxification pathways in the liver. Finally, bitter foods and herbs have been shown to boost metabolism, inhibit fat absorption, and prevent insulin spikes.

SIMPLE WAYS TO EAT THE DAISY FAMILY:

1. Toss wilted *escarole lettuce* in harissa paste and serve alongside roast chicken or broiled fish.

2. Prepare *Belgian endive* leaf cups with chopped walnuts and crumbled blue cheese to serve with an apéritif before dinner.

3. Marinate thinly sliced zucchini in olive oil, lemon juice, and chopped herbs for several hours, then arrange on a platter and garnish with bits of dressed *frisée*, pickled red onions, and lemon zest.

4. For a barbecue, cut small heads of *butter lettuce* in half, brush with oil and grill for 2 to 3 minutes before drizzling with a crème fraîche, chive, and lemon dressing.

5. Heat some oil in a pan, add cooked beans (such as cannellini), and fry until crispy before adding some garlic, *dandelion leaves*, and salt. As soon as the greens have wilted, drizzle with extra-virgin olive oil, and serve.

6. Mix different leaves such as loose-leaf, baby *cos* and *radicchio*, and dress with a shallot vinaigrette to serve alongside a rich meal.

7. Roughly chop *romaine lettuce* and toss with chunks of apple, pecan nuts and a tangy yogurt dressing, for a refreshing autumnal salad.

8. Cut *romaine lettuces* in half and spread salsa verde over the surface before roasting in a medium-hot oven for about 10 minutes, until the lettuce is slightly browned around the edges.

9. Toss *curly endive* with hot, roasted squash, finely chopped chives, olive oil, apple cider vinegar, and raisins, for a delicious side dish.

10. Cut heads of *Belgian endive* in half, drizzle with oil, season with salt and pepper, and roast in a hot oven for 15 minutes, then top with orange slices and soft goat cheese, before returning to the oven for another 15–20 minutes, or until tender and golden.

Herbs

What would our culinary world be like without these fragrant plants?! I rely heavily on these green leaves and stems to flavor food, but I also cherish herbs for their medicinal value and even to enliven closets and linens. Traditionally, different regions use specific varieties of herbs, and so a particular combination of flavors will frequently elicit memories of a country once visited or an exotic meal enjoyed. The leaves of many herbs can be dried and used as a substitute for fresh, but they often lose some intensity and create a more earthy flavor rather than provide a hit of freshness. Here are a few more commonly known culinary herbs and ideas for how to use them:

BASIL

A versatile and popular aromatic herb, basil is most often used in Mediterranean and Asian dishes, such as the classic pesto Genovese (made with basil, pine nuts, Parmesan or Pecorino cheese, and olive oil), or a Thai curry made with holy basil (tulsi). If you are a keen gardener, try growing some varieties with interesting flavors, such as pineapple, lemon, clove, and anise.

BAY LEAVES

I usually have a large bag of bay leaves at the ready to add whenever I cook grains, legumes, or large batches of stocks, soups, sauces, and stews. The bittersweet and mildly spicy leaves are best used when cooking times are slightly longer and, together with parsley and thyme, it forms part of the *bouquet garni* added to many classic French recipes. It is one of the few herbs that is equally good fresh or dried.

CHIVES

Chives are top greens in the allium family, which also includes garlic, scallions (the top greens of immature onions), and leeks. The long, thin and hollow green blades have a mild, grassy flavor and combine perfectly with chervil, parsley, and tarragon in the classic French blend known as *fines herbes*. Allium vegetables have been cultivated for centuries, not only for their invaluable pungent flavor, but also for their health benefits. Just like other allium members, chives possess thiosulfinate antioxidants, which convert to allicin—an organosulfur compound—by enzymatic reaction when its leaves are cut, chopped, or crushed. Studies have found that allicin, which has antibacterial, antiviral, and antifungal properties, is most potent directly after the cell membranes have been disturbed, and that heat destroys it. Allicin has also been found to help reduce cholesterol production, blood pressure, and overall risk of coronary artery disease, peripheral vascular diseases, and stroke.

CILANTRO

Cilantro (coriander) is the only herb I know of that elicits a "love or hate" response, but it is nonetheless used commonly across the world. Its tender stems and vibrant green leaves, not dissimilar in appearance to flat-leaf parsley, have a fresh, citrus taste, and very strong aroma. Leaf cilantro is best added to a dish just before serving, but coriander seeds (the dried berries) can withstand heat and longer cooking times. Cilantro is very rich in phytonutrients and antioxidants. Its leaves and seeds contain various essential oils and the plant is considered to be an antiseptic, analgesic, aphrodisiac, digestive aid, fungicide, and natural stimulant. It is also a very good source of vitamins A, C, K, and traces of the B vitamins, and calcium, potassium, iron, manganese, and sodium.

DILL

This green herb, with its wiry, threadlike leaves, has been used for culinary and medicinal purposes for hundreds of years. Like cilantro, the seeds can also be used. Dill's distinctive, slightly bitter taste is a combination of anise (or licorice), fennel, and celery. Dill's unique medicinal value is ascribed to mainly two healing components, namely monoterpenes—phytonutrients that exhibit an aromatic ring—and flavonoids, but it is also rich in minerals and certain amino acids. The health benefits of dill include its ability to boost digestive health, as well as provide relief from insomnia, hiccups, diarrhea, dysentery, menstrual disorders, respiratory disorders, and cancer. It is also good for oral care, can be a powerful boost for the immune system, and can protect from bone degradation. It is also an anti-inflammatory substance, so it can protect against arthritis, and relieve flatulence.

MARJORAM

Sweet marjoram—valued for centuries for its culinary and medicinal uses—is one of the most popular herbs used throughout the Mediterranean region. It is delicate and slightly sweet-tasting with a subtle pungency. In the US it is often referred to as, and confused with its bolder cousin, oregano. Marjoram is very effective in the treatment of coughs and colds. It is considered a potent decongestant and helps fight viral infection, bronchitis, sinusitis, and sinus headaches. It is also believed to have a calming effect and support cardiac health due to its flavonoid content, and is a wonderful aid in digestion-related disorders.

MINT

The herb often associated with a fresh breath is also a very versatile kitchen companion. Of the two dozen species, the one grown and used most widely is spearmint, but peppermint, with its darker green leaves and sharper flavor, is also used, mainly to flavor confectionery and ice cream. Mint has antiseptic qualities, aids digestion (by activating the salivary and digestive enzyme glands), and is known to soothe respiratory complaints. I particularly like mint for its ability to naturally uplift and stimulate when I am having a low point.

OREGANO (OR WILD MARJORAM)

I have used oregano several times in the recipes in this book, as it is really delicious and has some wonderful health benefits. Origanum bushes produce strong stems with dark-green leaves that have a pungent, slightly floral and bitter taste with citrus undertones. This herb loves garlic and lamb, and can hold its own when combined with vinegar or lemon. Like most herbs, oregano has a much higher antioxidant level than other fruit and vegetables, and is also rich in vitamins and minerals. Additionally, oregano contains potent antimicrobial phytochemicals, and has some antiviral properties.

PARSLEY

This is my favorite multitasker. Even though it has a distinct flavor, it is strangely neutral and manages to blend in with many foods and flavors. I often toss a handful into my smoothie and whenever I feel a meal lacks chlorophyll, I add a huge amount of finely chopped parsley. There are two main varieties: curly-leaf and flat-leaf, with the latter having a slightly stronger taste. Parsley belongs to the *Apiaceae* family, along with carrots, celery, and other herbs like cumin, dill, lovage, angelica, and anise.
The herb contains valuable volatile oils and flavonoids that have chemo-protective benefits and act as antioxidants to protect cells from oxidative damage and stress. The herb is also antibacterial, anti-inflammatory, and a great source of vitamin C and beta-carotene (pro-vitamin A).

ROSEMARY

We have a huge rosemary bush in our garden and I run out for twigs regularly throughout the year. The pine needlelike leaves are a versatile flavoring agent that can be used in a vast number of dishes. Add the whole stem to a pot roast or strip the leaves off and chop them up very finely before including in a wintry pasta dish. Rosemary has also been used as a natural remedy for a variety of ailments over the centuries. It has powerful antioxidant, anti-inflammatory, antibacterial, and anticarcinogenic properties, is said to improve memory, lift mood, relieve migraines and pain in general, detoxify the liver, and help treat digestive problems. It can also be used as a natural remedy for respiratory problems.

SAGE

Native to the Mediterranean and Balkans, sage is a member of the mint family and has a very strong, musty, slightly bitter flavor, so use with care. Sage leaves are grayish-green (sometimes purple) and velvety, and can withstand long cooking times. In fact, sage is very rarely eaten raw. Often used with poultry, sage seems to go especially well with fatty dishes and is believed to aid in their digestion. Its antiseptic and astringent properties make sage ideal for many conditions of the mouth and throat, and it is also said to improve memory.

TARRAGON

Often used in French cooking (it is one of the herbs that makes up *fines herbes* and is used in Béarnaise sauce), this herb has long, soft, bright-green leaves and an aniseed flavor with a hint of vanilla. A perfect match for poultry, fish, eggs, and cheese, use fresh or dried tarragon to flavor dishes, sauces, or condiments. This herb has been used by numerous cultures for centuries as a natural treatment for many ailments (such as toothache and digestive issues), and is high in vitamins, potassium, and other nutrients that have been proven to provide health benefits.

THYME

Another member of the mint family, subtle thyme (in all its varieties) is an essential component of any cook's arsenal. It grows in long, thin sprigs with small green leaves, which are mostly stripped from the stalk, although whole sprigs can also be added to dishes such as stews, soups, and sauces, and removed before serving. It pairs well with other Mediterranean herbs like oregano and marjoram, and is used throughout Italian, French, and Mediterranean cooking. Just like the other herbs, thyme is packed with health-promoting components. Among others it supports eye health, helps cure coughs and colds, has antibacterial properties, helps control blood pressure, improves bone health, and aids digestion.

SIMPLE WAYS TO EAT HERBS:

1. Toast fresh *oregano* leaves lightly in a pan before adding them to your favorite chili con carne recipe.

2. Sprinkle fresh whole leaves of *marjoram* in a salad of greens.

3. Put fresh *tarragon* sprigs and peeled garlic cloves into a sterilized bottle with cider vinegar. Place in a dark spot for a few days and remove the sprigs once the desired strength has been reached.

4. Wrap several *rosemary* twigs in some cheesecloth and add to a pot of beans while they are cooking. You will impart the flavor without having to pick out hundreds of needles.

5. Sprinkle *oregano* leaves over cubes of goat milk feta and mixed olives, then drizzle with olive oil.

6. Finely shred fresh *mint* and add to chocolate chip cookie dough.

7. Toss *marjoram* and toasted pecans with thinly sliced oranges and leeks dressed with pecan oil.

8. Add fresh *thyme* leaves to a marinade for vegetable kebabs at your next barbecue.

9. One of the best uses for *oregano* in your cooking is adding it to a dry rub or a marinade for meat (that includes cloves, cinnamon, rosemary, ginger, black pepper, paprika, garlic) prior to cooking, which may help reduce the toxic compounds created during the cooking process.

10. For a great snack, place a fresh anchovy between two *sage* leaves and fry in some hot oil until crisp.

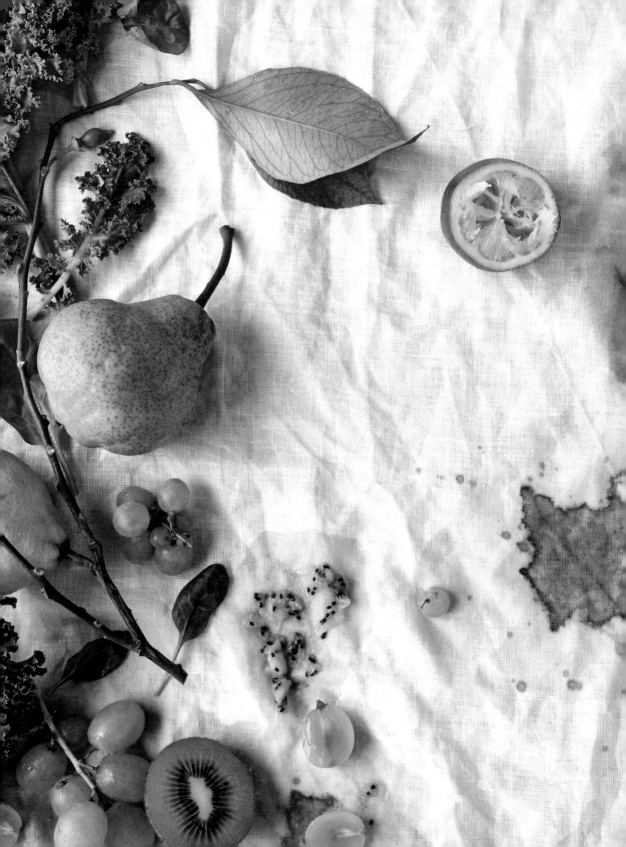

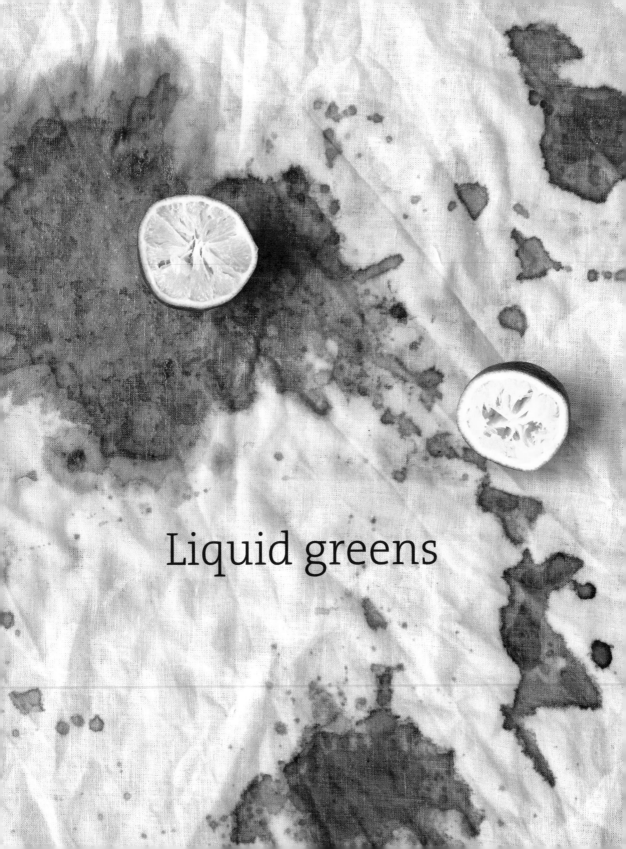

Liquid greens

Juices/smoothies

- Aim to use more vegetables than fruit when preparing fresh juices. Make this shift gradually if you are new to juicing.

- Freshly pressed vegetable juices are a useful way of increasing nutrient intake, especially in those with digestive problems or other health issues.

- Freshly juiced tonics should be consumed as soon as possible after making, as exposure to light and oxygen starts degrading the juice at once.

- Buy produce that's been minimally sprayed with pesticides, as you are using the whole fruit or veg.

- Vegetable juices should be seen as a nutrient supplement under normal circumstances and not as a meal replacement unless you are following a juice-based detox for a few days. Smoothies, on the other hand, are akin to a (liquid) meal, so bear this in mind when you have a large smoothie and feel entitled to a fry-up, too!

- To increase nutrient absorption:
  1. Drink green juices on an empty stomach or two hours after having eaten, and wait at least 20 minutes before eating your next meal
  2. Consume some fat with juices and smoothies (liquid coconut oil, nuts, or nut butters and seeds)
  3. Drink juices and smoothies at room temperature —it is kinder on your digestion
  4. Always include a vitamin C-rich food (such as lemon or lime) in your green juice and smoothie, or have some soon after, as this helps reduce the effect of the oxalic acid or antinutrients found in many leafy greens (such as spinach and chard)

- Alternate greens frequently. Regular consumption of raw cruciferous vegetables, for example, may affect those with thyroid dysfunction due to the goitrogens.

- Always start juicing with the leafy greens and herbs, followed by the soft fruits and ginger, and lastly any chunky produce such as apple, carrot, celery, or cucumber, to help the juicer do its job.

- Chew your drinks and drink your food! If you don't swirl the drink around in your mouth and chew a few times, the digestive process, which starts with saliva production in the mouth and a signal being sent to the brain to release digestive juices in the stomach, is compromised.

Juices
ALL SERVE 2 TO 3

1. Citrus green

Very refreshing and just like a cold citron pressé, only bright green.

7oz (200g) kale (stalks and leaves)

Small handful of parsley

1 cucumber

1 lemon, partially peeled (leave about one-fifth of the skin on)

1 lime, peeled

2 green apples (or red ones for a sweeter taste)

Wash all the ingredients well and chop into manageable chunks, then juice in the order listed. Stir and serve.

2. Lettuce and pear

7oz (200g) cos or other crunchy leaf lettuce

Large handful of basil leaves

2 ripe pears

1 lime, partially peeled (leave about half the skin on)

1 satsuma, mandarin, or tangerine, peeled

Wash all the ingredients well and chop into manageable chunks, then juice in the order listed. You may want to pass the juice through a strainer to filter out any soft pulp that might have slipped through. Otherwise, it will be a little thicker than a regular juice. Stir and serve.

3. Collard greens, pineapple, and ginger

I love the spiciness the cabbage greens add to this juice, but it might not be the easiest way to get your family drinking green juices, so feel free to replace the collard greens with other greens of your choice.

5¼oz (150g) collard greens or green cabbage, tough stalks removed, coarsely chopped

½ cucumber

1 orange, partially peeled (leave about one-fifth of the skin on)

½ ripe pineapple, peeled

½-in (1-cm) piece ginger (large if you like it spicy)

½ lemon, peeled

Wash all the ingredients well and chop into manageable chunks, then juice in the order listed. Stir and serve.

4. Lamb's lettuce, green grape, and kiwi

7oz (200g) lamb's lettuce (mâche) or baby spinach leaves

Large handful of mint leaves

1 cup (150g) green grapes

3 kiwi fruit, unpeeled

½ cucumber

1 celery stalk

Wash all the ingredients well and chop into manageable chunks, then juice in the order listed.

Either give the juice a quick whizz in a blender for an ultrasmooth, thick juice, or pass it through a strainer to filter out any soft pulp that may have slipped through. Stir and serve.

Nettle and dandelion infusion

Both nettle tips and dandelion leaves are renowned for their medicinal properties and should be available in select healthfood stores or ethnic grocers. I always have different infusion blends on the shelf to offer my guests, be it for their relaxing, immune-boosting or energizing properties.
MAKES ENOUGH FOR ROUGHLY 15 CUPS OF TEA

½oz (15g) dried nettle leaves

½oz (15g) dried dandelion leaves

¼oz (10g) dried peppermint leaves

2 Tbsp fennel seeds, crushed with mortar and pestle or partially ground in a spice grinder

⅛oz (5g) dried red rose petals

Mix all the ingredients together well and store in an airtight container.

To make a single serving of the infusion, put 1 heaping Tbsp of the loose leaf tea in a teapot and pour 1 to 1¼ cups (250 to 300ml) boiling water over. Let steep for 2 to 3 minutes, then pour through a strainer to enjoy.

ALL JUICES PHOTOGRAPHED ON PAGES 22 TO 23

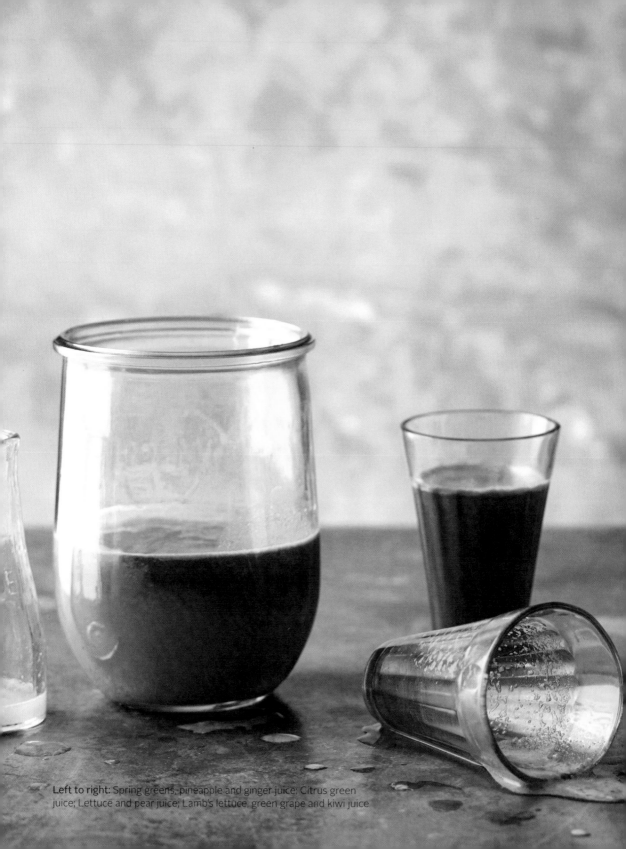

Left to right: Spring greens, pineapple and ginger juice; Citrus green juice; Lettuce and pear juice; Lamb's lettuce, green grape and kiwi juice

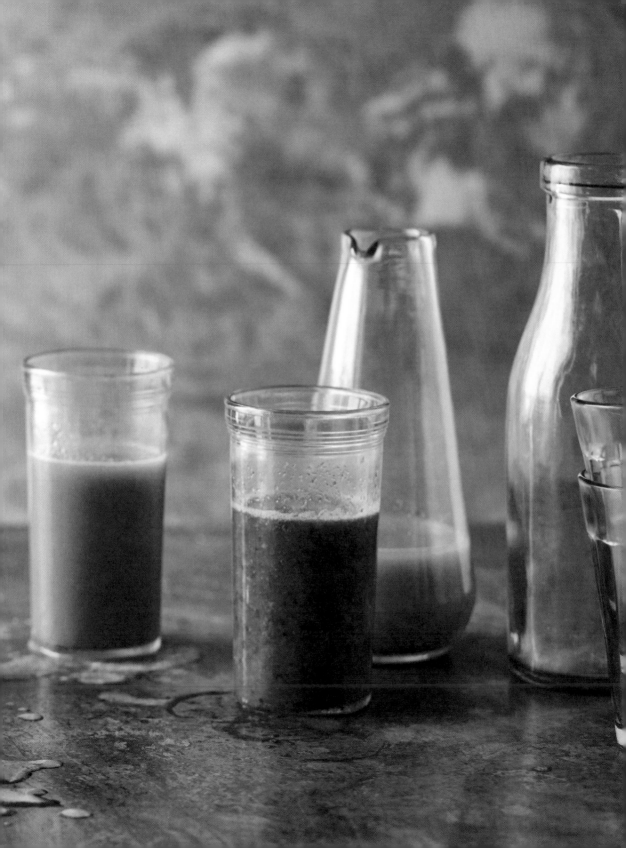

Smoothies

ALL SERVE 2 TO 3

1. The Pick-me-up

This is a good choice when you need rehydration and energy. Rooibos (redbush) tea, dried figs, blueberries, and chia seeds are all rich in antioxidants, and figs contain more fiber than any other fruit. Lamb's lettuce is packed with Vitamin B9, known for its antifatigue and antistress properties. It is also very rich in eye-protecting Vitamin A and multitasking Vitamin B6. To top it off, it has almost as high an iron content as spinach, but is very low in oxalates, which prevent nutrients from being absorbed.

1 cup (250ml) strong rooibos tea, cooled

1 tsp chia seeds

2 large dried figs, coarsely chopped

1 large very ripe banana, cut or broken into chunks

½ tsp good-quality vanilla extract

Large handful (about 1oz/30g) lamb's lettuce (mâche)

1¼ cups (150g) frozen (or fresh) blueberries

Juice of 1 lime

Prepare the tea the night before.

Pour the cooled tea into the blender and add the chia seeds. Stir a few times while you get the rest of your ingredients together.

Now add everything else, including the blueberries, and blend until smooth.

2. Ultimate green

If you are not one for green smoothies in general, you should try this one. It is quite delicious and very virtuous. It helps having a high-speed blender, but if you don't, just keep blending until the mixture is smooth. You will need to soak the almonds overnight, and if you struggle to buy frozen mango or pineapple, peel and chop up the fruit the night before and freeze it.

1 lemon

1½ cups (375ml) coconut water, preferably raw

⅜-in (1-cm) piece ginger, peeled and coarsely chopped

Handful of almonds, soaked overnight, or for at least 6 hours, and rinsed

Big handful of kale, thick stalks discarded, leaves coarsely chopped or torn

1 tsp green powder of your choice (optional)

1 ripe medium banana, cut or broken into chunks

1½ to 1¾ cups (200 to 220g) frozen fruit

Cut the lemon in half then cut a thick slice off one half. Chop this up roughly and place in a blender. Squeeze the juice from the remaining lemon halves and add, together with the coconut water, ginger, and almonds, to the blender. Blend until smooth.

Add the rest of the ingredients and blend until smooth and creamy. If your blender allows for the use of a tamper, it is a good idea to press the frozen fruits down into the blade to avoid uneven blending.

3. Pumpkin pie

According to my husband, this smoothie has it all. It's a great way to use up leftover butternut squash, pumpkin, or sweet potato and is a wonderful breakfast or late-afternoon snack.

Finely grated zest of 1 small orange

1 cup (250ml) fresh orange juice (about 3 oranges) (or half milk of your choice, and half orange juice)

½ small Dolce Verde romaine lettuce heart, trimmed and coarsely chopped

2 pitted large Medjool dates

3oz (80g) cooked butternut squash (or pumpkin or sweet potato)

1 Tbsp peanut (or other nut) butter

Large pinch of ground cinnamon

A few pinches of freshly grated nutmeg

Handful of ice cubes

Blend the orange zest, juice, lettuce, and dates until smooth. Add the rest of the ingredients, except the ice cubes, and blend until smooth. Add the ice and blend one last time until smooth.

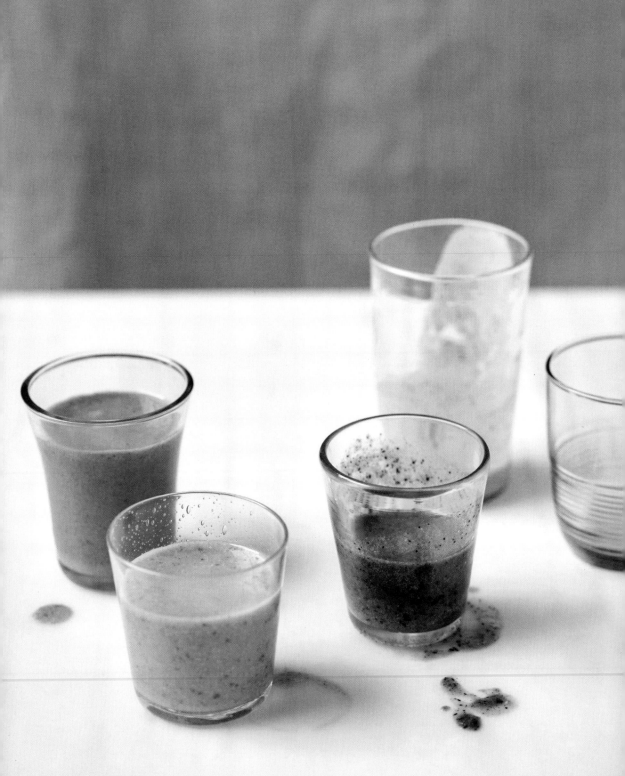

Left to right, from back: Pumpkin pie smoothie;
Ultimate green smoothie; The pick-me-up smoothie

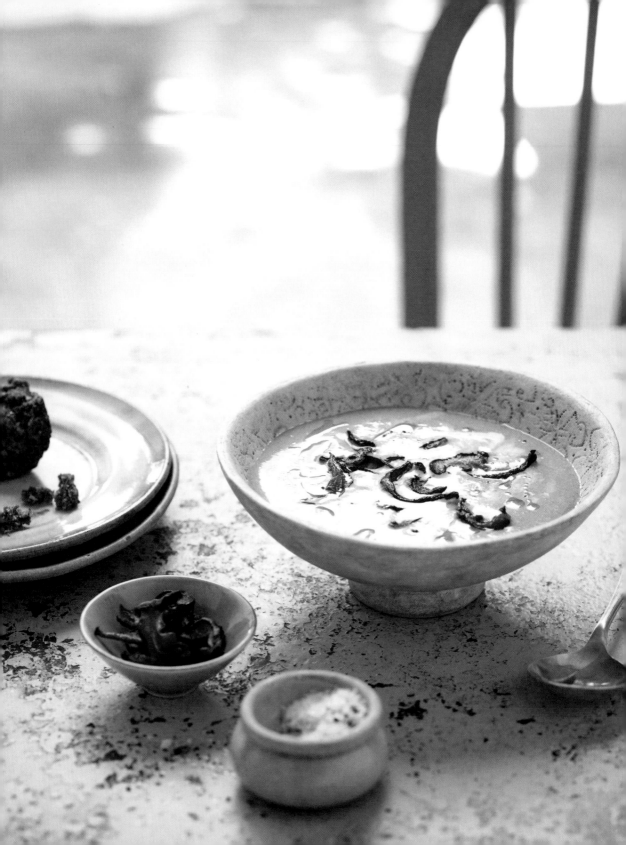

Creamy Tuscan kale and shiitake mushroom soup

I love this one. It is perhaps not surprising that it tastes wonderful, given the added cream, but if you are able to find unpasteurized dairy from pastured animals, it needn't be a guilty pleasure, especially as both Tuscan kale (also called lacinato, cavolo nero, or black cabbage) and shiitakes are considered extremely health-supportive. For the crispy shiitake, use large mushrooms, as they shrink considerably while baking. SERVES 4

Carefully toss the mushrooms for the crispy shiitake with the salt and smoked paprika, then spread out in a single layer on a baking tray lined with baking parchment. Drizzle with the olive oil, ensuring most mushrooms receive some. Let stand for at least 15 minutes to allow the spices to penetrate. Meanwhile, preheat the oven to 320°F (160°C).

Bake the mushrooms for 20 to 30 minutes or until they have shrunk considerably and are crispy around the edges, rotating the baking tray once during cooking and keeping an eye on them toward the end to avoid burning. Remove from the oven and set aside to cool.

Meanwhile, put the dried mushrooms in a small bowl and add enough warm water to cover. Let soak for 15 minutes.

Gently heat the oil in a large saucepan, add the onion, and sweat over low heat for a few minutes until soft and translucent. Add the sliced fresh shiitakes and fry over relatively high heat until cooked and slightly caramelized.

Add the soaked mushrooms with their liquid, the Tuscan kale, sweet potato, and broth, and simmer for about 20 minutes until the sweet potato is tender.

Blend the soup until smooth and velvety, then return it to the pan and stir in nearly all the cream, keeping some back to serve. Keep the soup hot, but don't let it boil once the cream has been added.

Season with lemon juice, salt, and black pepper, and serve with a drizzle of porcini oil, a splash of cream, and the crispy shiitake.

⅓ cup (10g) dried wild mushrooms

Splash of extra-virgin olive oil

1 medium onion, coarsely chopped

4¼oz (125g) fresh shiitake mushrooms, stems removed, sliced

5 cups (200g) Tuscan kale, thick stems removed, coarsely chopped

1 medium sweet potato, peeled and cut into large dice

2 cups (500ml) vegetable or fresh chicken broth

Generous 2 cups (500ml) light cream (cow, goat, or sheep), plus extra for garnish

Squeeze of lemon juice, to taste

Sea salt and freshly ground black pepper

Porcini oil, to serve

FOR THE CRISPY SHIITAKE
4¼oz (125g) large fresh shiitake mushrooms, stems removed, thinly sliced

Pinch of fine sea salt

1 tsp smoked paprika

1 Tbsp olive oil

Collard greens and smoked haddock soup with watercress snow

This is a very hearty, warming soup and definitely a proper meal-in-one. It is also quite kid-friendly, and easy to prepare in advance up to the step of adding the fish. The watercress snow makes enough to serve 8, but the surplus will keep well in the freezer for at least a couple of months. You need to make it the day before, to allow for freezing time. SERVES 4

In a small food processor, blitz all the ingredients, except the olive oil, for the watercress snow, scraping down the sides a few times, then stir in the olive oil until it just reaches a saucelike consistency.

Transfer to a flat, shallow container and place in the freezer for at least 6 hours.

When you are ready to make the soup, heat the oil or butter in a large saucepan over medium heat, add the leek, celery, onions, and garlic with a pinch of salt and sweat until soft and translucent. Add the potatoes and cook a little longer, resisting the urge to stir.

Add the broth, wine, ground fennel, and bay leaves, and bring to a boil. Reduce the heat and simmer for about 20 minutes with the lid ajar until the potatoes are tender.

Remove the bay leaves and blend the soup until smooth. Add salt and pepper to taste, and a little hot water if it is too thick. Return the soup to the pan and stir in the greens. Simmer until tender, then either remove half the soup and blend again, or use a stick blender to partially blend the soup in the pan; you want a smooth soup with bits of greens to chew on.

Add the fish and simmer for a few minutes until it is cooked through or flaky. Be careful not to overcook it, as it will become dry and stringy.

While the fish is cooking, remove the watercress snow from the freezer and cut half into chunks (return the rest to the freezer for another occasion). Process the chunks in a blender to make a frozen powder, or use a sharp knife to chop it up.

Serve the soup hot with lots of watercress snow and the reserved toasted, chopped almonds.

A little olive or coconut oil, or butter

1 leek, trimmed, sliced in half lengthwise and sliced across into half-moons

2 celery stalks, trimmed and coarsely chopped

2 medium onions (about 7oz/200g), coarsely chopped

2 large garlic cloves, coarsely chopped

2 large potatoes (about 14oz/400g), peeled and cut into medium dice

4½ cups (1L) fish or vegetable broth

½ cup (125ml) dry white wine (or extra broth)

1 tsp fennel seeds, toasted in dry frying pan for 1 to 2 minutes until fragrant, then finely ground

2 bay leaves

2 cups (300g/1 medium bunch) collard greens, very finely shredded

10½oz (300g) undyed smoked haddock fillet, cut into bite-size pieces

Sea salt and freshly ground black pepper

FOR THE WATERCRESS SNOW
3½oz (100g) watercress

½ cup (60g) almonds, toasted in hot oven for 7 to 8 minutes (set aside half for garnish)

Squeeze of lemon juice

1 garlic clove, finely chopped

Pinch each of sea salt and freshly ground black pepper

1 to 2 Tbsp extra-virgin olive oil

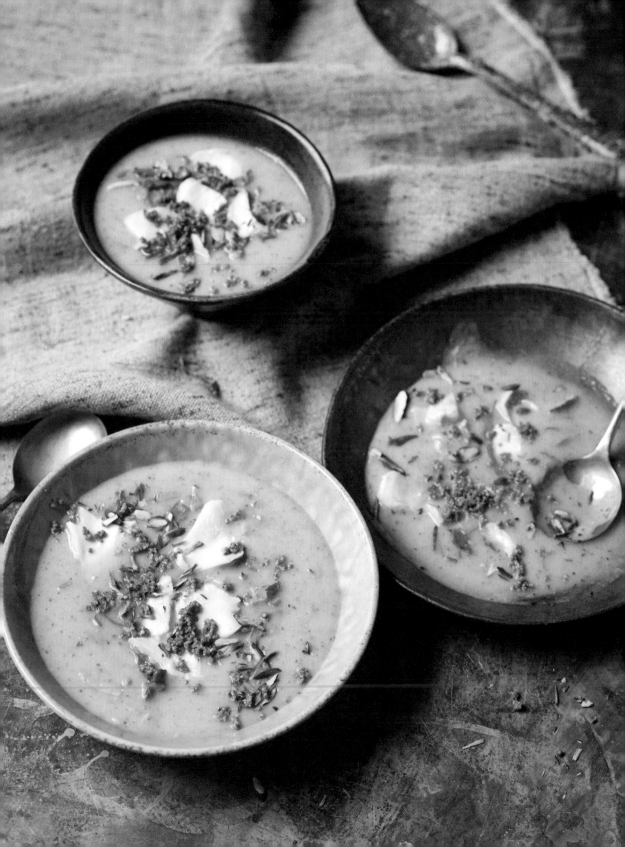

Green gazpacho

Gazpacho always reminds me of the disappointed look on my dad's face the first time he had this traditional Spanish soup. He loves all things tomato, but did not expect something cold ... Since then we have all grown to love cold soups during the hot summer months. They are wonderful for entertaining, as they can be prepared in advance. If you have more ripe avocados than you need here, dice them, toss with lime juice, and sprinkle over the soup before adding the ice cubes. Another option is to serve it with chopped chives or dill and a dollop of sour cream. SERVES 4

Start preparing this recipe the day before you intend to serve this soup. For the ice cubes, juice the cucumber (or blend and strain through a nut milk bag or several layers of cheesecloth), then stir in the lime juice and season generously with salt and pepper. Fill each cavity of the ice tray with the cucumber juice, then place a small edible flower or mint leaf in each. Freeze overnight. The dark green bits will sink to the bottom, creating a beautiful color contrast when the cubes start to melt in each bowl of soup.

The next day, juice the cucumbers, celery, apple, and scallions. Alternatively, you could use a powerful blender and strain the pulp through a few layers of cheesecloth or a nut milk bag.

Transfer to a clean blender, add the lime juice and avocados, and blend until smooth. Add the Worcestershire sauce with Tabasco, lemon juice, salt, and pepper to taste.

Serve on a hot day with a few cucumber ice cubes added to each serving.

2 large cucumbers, peeled and coarsely chopped

2 celery stalks, chopped

1 large green apple, chopped

2 scallions, cut into quarters

Juice of 1 to 2 limes, to taste

2 small avocados (about 8¾oz/250g), peeled and cubed

1 Tbsp Worcestershire sauce

Tabasco, to taste

Squeeze of lemon juice

Sea salt and freshly ground black pepper

FOR THE ICE CUBES
1 cucumber

Juice of 1 lime

Edible flowers, such as borage, or small mint leaves

Sea salt and black pepper

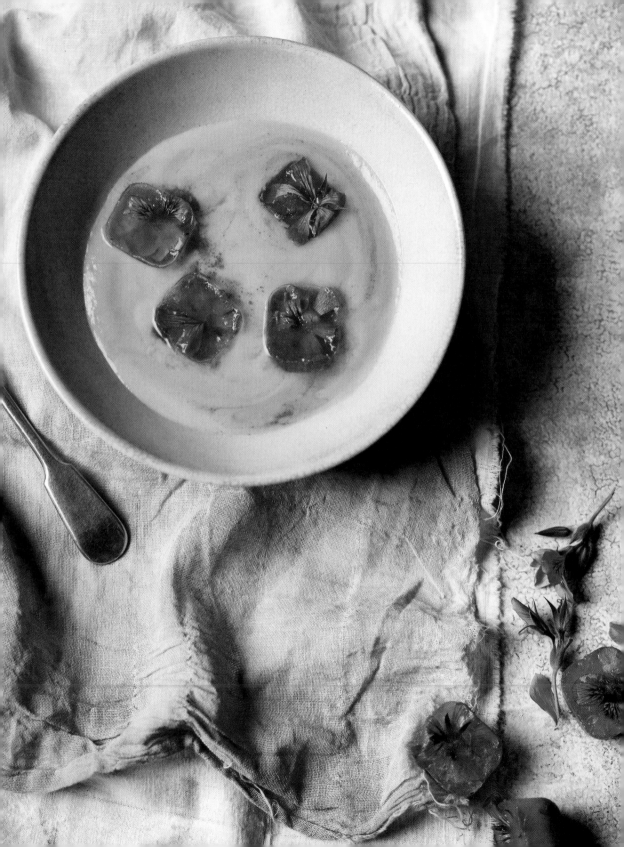

Pumpkin and tamarind soup

This is a delicious North African-inspired soup that would make a great appetizer course, but is equally good as a light meal with some flatbread and hummus. Tamarinds are tart fruits often used as a spice and souring agent in South Asian, but also North African, dishes. They are rich in tartaric acid (a powerful antioxidant), several minerals and vitamins, and contain many volatile phytochemicals with medicinal properties. SERVES 4

Heat a little coconut oil in a large saucepan and brown the diced pumpkin in batches. You are looking for some caramelization on the surfaces.

Put all the pumpkin back into the pan with the garlic, leek, and ginger and sauté for another couple of minutes, taking care not to burn the garlic.

Now add the broth and tamarind paste and simmer for 5 to 10 minutes, or until the pumpkin is just tender. Add the bok choy stalks and continue to cook until these, too, are tender.

Remove the pan from the heat and add the orange juice. Blend until smooth using a blender or stick blender. Stir in the chopped cilantro. Keep warm, but don't let boil.

For the spice oil, heat the coconut oil in a small saucepan until hot but not smoking. Add the mustard seeds and fry until they start to pop (a couple of minutes). Add the red pepper flakes and cumin seeds and cook until fragrant (another couple of minutes). Add the ground coriander and turmeric and cook for a minute longer.

Lastly, stir the bok choy leaves and most of the spice oil into the hot soup, and serve garnished with a sprig of fresh cilantro and a drizzle of spice oil.

Coconut oil, for frying

2½lb (1.2kg) pumpkin (or butternut squash), peeled and cut into large cubes (should yield 2 to 2¼lb/900g to 1kg)

2 large garlic cloves, finely chopped

1 leek, trimmed, halved lengthwise, and sliced into half-moons

1 heaping Tbsp freshly grated ginger

2½ to 2⅔ cups (580 to 625ml) vegetable or fresh chicken broth

2 Tbsp tart tamarind paste

10½oz (300g) bok choy, stalks and leaves separate

Juice of 1 orange (about 3 Tbsp)

Small bunch of fresh cilantro, finely chopped (set aside a few sprigs to garnish)

FOR THE SPICE OIL

2 Tbsp coconut oil

2 tsp yellow mustard seeds

½ to 1 tsp dried red pepper flakes (or more, to taste)

3 tsp cumin seeds

3 tsp ground coriander

1 tsp ground turmeric

Spinach, broccoli and lentil soup with Stilton croutons

Green vegetables are so beautiful when pureed or blended! They owe their vibrant color to chlorophyll, a green pigment instrumental in the process of photosynthesis that has many health benefits when consumed. Usually the color starts to become faded after exposure to heat for more than 10 minutes. So, to ensure your soup retains its glorious hue, I suggest cooking the lentils separately first, but if this is too much of a faff, just add them to the soup after you have blended it. SERVES 4

Soak the lentils in four times their volume of cold water for at least 6 hours, or overnight.

Preheat the oven to 320°F (160°C). If using bacon, place a wire rack inside a lipped baking sheet and lay the bacon slices on top. Bake in the oven for 20 to 30 minutes, until crispy around the edges. Remove them using tongs, blot any excess fat with paper towels, cut into small strips, and set aside.

For the croutons, toss the bread cubes in a little olive oil, season with salt and pepper, and place closely together on a lipped baking sheet. Sprinkle over the crumbled blue cheese, being careful to keep most of the cheese on the bread and not on the sheet. Bake for 15 minutes or until crunchy, then remove from the oven and let cool.

If cooking the lentils separately (see Introduction above), drain them and put into a small saucepan with double their volume of fresh water, the garlic clove, and bay leaf. Bring to a boil, then reduce the heat, cover, and simmer for 15 minutes or until they are just tender.

Meanwhile, heat the oil in a soup pan and gently cook the leeks, celery, and broccoli stems until just tender, 5 to 10 minutes, depending on thickness.

Add the broccoli florets, most of the broth (setting some aside to adjust the consistency of the soup at the end), and all the spices. Simmer, uncovered, for about 5 minutes until all the vegetables are tender.

Stir in half the spinach and remove from the heat as soon as it has wilted. Blend the soup with the remaining spinach until completely smooth.

Return to the pan and add the lentils. If you didn't cook the lentils separately, simmer, uncovered, for another 15 minutes, or until lentils are just cooked. Adjust the seasoning and add a little more broth if the soup is too thick.

Stir in the bacon, if using, and serve topped with cheesy croutons.

½ cup (100g) dried green lentils

7oz (200g) unsmoked bacon slices (optional)

1 garlic clove, crushed, and 1 bay leaf (only if cooking the lentils separately)

A glug of extra-virgin olive oil

2 medium leeks (about 14oz/400g), trimmed, halved lengthwise, and sliced into half-moons

3 celery stalks, trimmed and coarsely chopped

11¼ to 12oz (320 to 340g) broccoli, stem finely chopped and florets coarsely chopped

5 cups (1.2L) hot vegetable broth

Pinch of cayenne pepper

¼ tsp ground allspice

Seeds of 5 cardamom pods

4 cups (200g) spinach, washed

FOR THE CROUTONS
5¼ oz (150g) sourdough bread (2 to 3 thickish slices from a large loaf), cut into cubes

Extra-virgin olive oil

Scant ½ to ½ cup (50 to 60g) stilton or other blue-veined cheese, crumbled

Sea salt and freshly ground black pepper

Watercress, pea and corn soup with mint and onion popcorn

This is one of my absolute favorites, with the mountain of white popcorn gloriously set off against the greenest of greens. SERVES 4

Heat a tiny bit of butter, ghee, or olive oil in a saucepan and gently sweat the onion with a large pinch of salt until soft and translucent. Add the celery and cook for another few minutes before adding the garlic.

Cook for another minute or so, then add half the peas and half the corn kernels, with the split peas and broth. Bring to a boil, then reduce the heat and simmer gently for 20 to 25 minutes, until the split peas are tender.

While the soup is cooking, make the popcorn. Heat the oil or butter in deep saucepan and sprinkle the popcorn over the bottom. Cover with a lid and wait for a few minutes until they start to pop.

Meanwhile, mix together the melted butter, salt, mint, and garlic powder. As soon as the popping has slowed down significantly, pour this mixture over the popcorn. Remove from the heat, cover with the lid, and give the pan a few good shakes. Set aside.

As soon as the split peas are tender, add the watercress and cook just until the leaves wilt. Remove from the heat and add the milk and mint leaves.

Blend until smooth, then return to the pan, stir in the remaining peas and corn, and season with salt and pepper. Reheat briefly and gently before serving.

Serve the soup in bowls topped with a mound of popcorn, some shredded mint, and the remaining spice crumbs from the bottom of the popcorn pan. Don't stir the popcorn into the soup as you eat it, as it will turn soggy and not be nearly as much fun to eat.

Butter, ghee or olive oil

1 medium onion, chopped

2 celery stalks (about 4oz/120g trimmed weight), coarsely chopped

1 large garlic clove, chopped

¾ cup (110g) peas, fresh or frozen

1 ear of corn, kernels sliced off

125g yellow split peas, rinsed

2⅔ to 3 cups (625 to 750ml) vegetable broth

200g watercress, leaves and stalks

1½ cups (375ml) whole milk or milk substitute, such as almond or coconut milk

Large handful of mint leaves

Sea salt and freshly ground black pepper

FOR THE POPCORN

1½ tsp coconut or canola oil, or butter

Scant ¼ cup (40g) popping corn, preferably organic

2 tsp melted butter

Pinch of sea salt

1 tsp finely shredded mint leaves, plus extra to serve

½ tsp dried garlic powder or granules

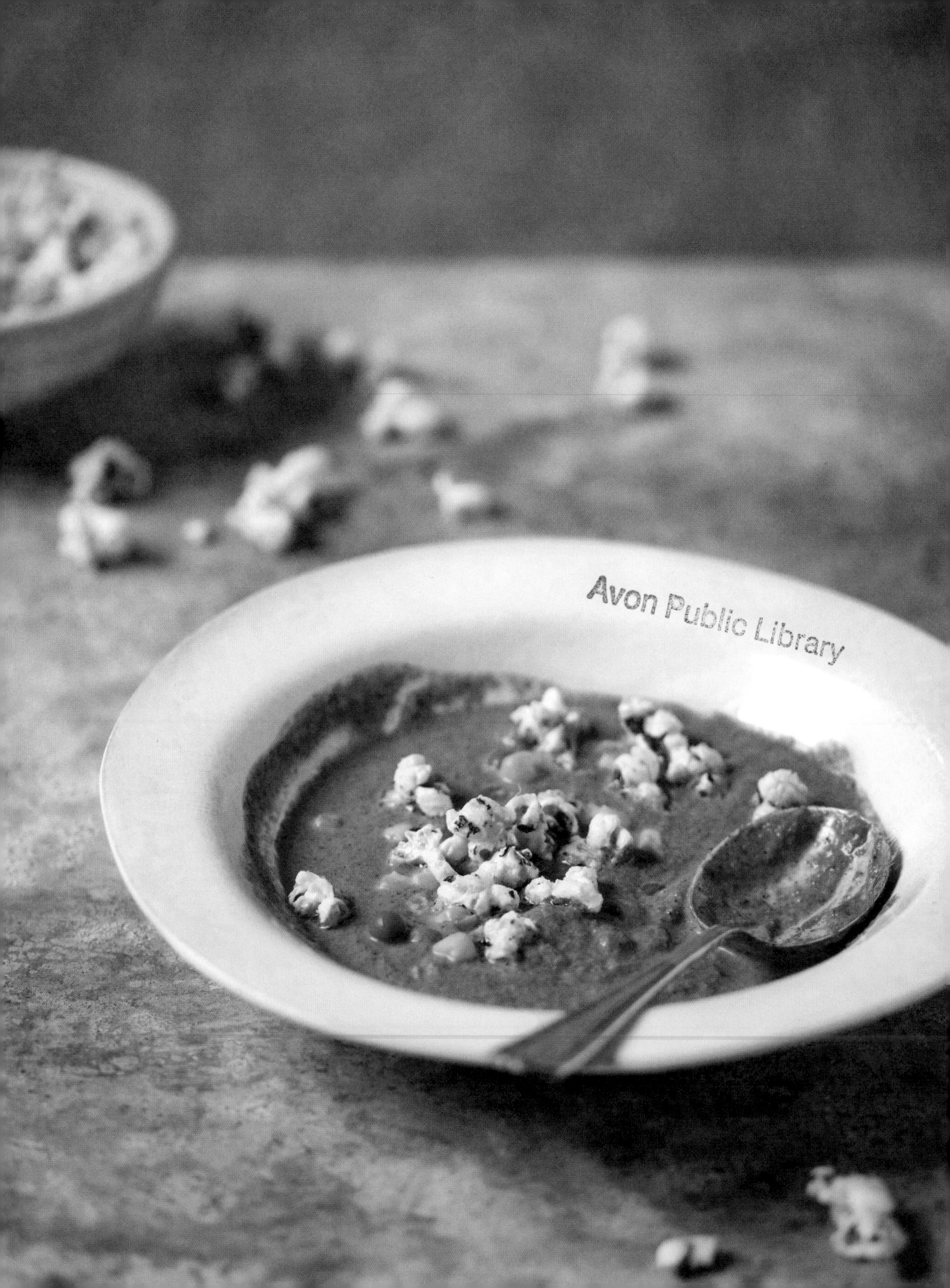

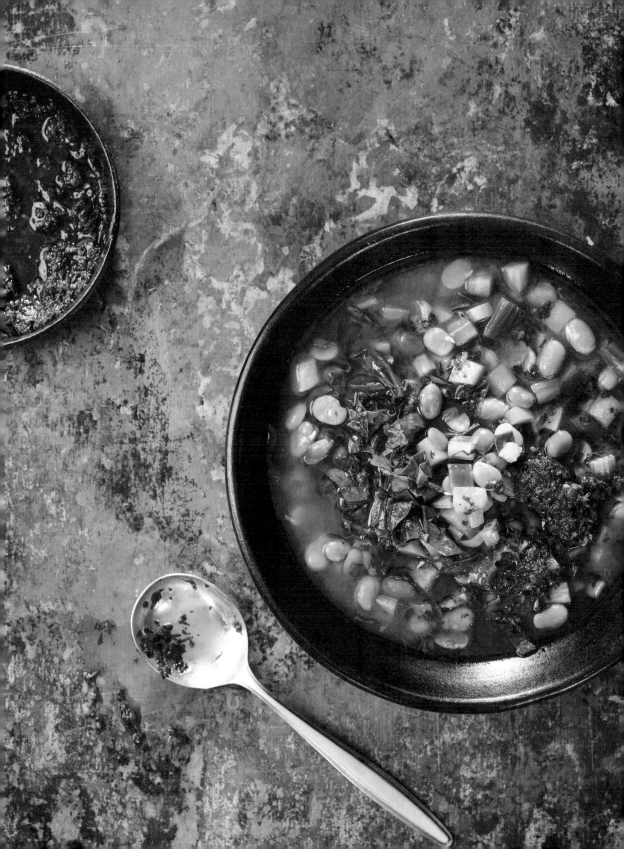

Rich tomato broth with chard, borlotti beans, and parsley pistou

This is a good example of a recipe that can be altered to suit your mood, available time, and audience. It seems complicated, but really doesn't take much time at all. You could blend the broth and the rest of the cooked vegetables for a thick and hearty vegetable soup, particularly good with some sour cream stirred through. The parsley pistou provides an essential hit of freshness and flavor. SERVES 4 TO 6

For the broth, gently heat the oil in a saucepan, add the onion, celery, and carrot with a large pinch of salt and cook for a few minutes until the onion is soft and translucent. Add the garlic and dried herbs and cook for another minute or two before adding the rest of the broth ingredients. Bring to a boil, reduce the heat slightly, and simmer, uncovered, for 30 minutes.

Meanwhile, for the soup, use a vegetable swivel peeler to remove the outer layer of the fennel bulb. Separate the bulb into layers and chop each layer into small dice.

When the broth is ready, let cool slightly before straining through a strainer. Use the back of a large metal or wooden spoon to press the vegetables down in the strainer and squeeze out every last bit of liquid, which will help to give the broth some body. Discard the pulp.

Return the broth to the pan, season with salt and pepper, then add the diced potatoes and carrot. Cover and simmer for about 5 minutes, or until the potatoes are very close to tender.

Add the fennel, chard stalks, and zucchini, cover, and simmer for another few minutes, or until the chard stalks are tender. Stir in the shredded chard leaves and simmer, uncovered, for a few minutes, before adding the fava beans or peas, with the cooked borlotti beans. Remove from the heat once the peas and borlotti beans are heated through. Do not leave on the heat for too long at this stage, or the greens and peas lose their lovely bright green color.

Serve immediately with a large dollop of Parsley Pistou and some sourdough toast.

1 quantity of Parsley Pistou (page 41)

FOR THE BROTH
2 Tbsp extra-virgin olive oil

1 onion, finely chopped

2 celery stalks, finely chopped

1 small carrot, scrubbed clean and finely chopped

2 garlic cloves, coarsely chopped

2 tsp dried marjoram or oregano

2¼ lb (1kg/about 8 large or 12 small) ripe tomatoes, fibrous core removed and coarsely chopped

2 tsp tomato paste

Large pinch of unrefined brown sugar

2 bay leaves

5 cups (1.2L) hot vegetable broth

Sea salt and freshly ground black pepper

FOR THE SOUP
12¼oz (350g) fennel (1 large bulb), trimmed

8¾ oz (250g/about 2 medium) potatoes, peeled and cut into small dice

5¼ oz (150g/about 1 medium to large) carrot, cut into small dice

7oz (200g) chard, stalks diced and leaves finely shredded

7 to 8½ oz (200 to 250g/1 large or 2 small) zucchini, cut into small dice

¾ cup (110g) baby or freshly picked fava beans, or peas

2 cups (280g) cooked borlotti beans (⅔cup/120g dried, see page 152)

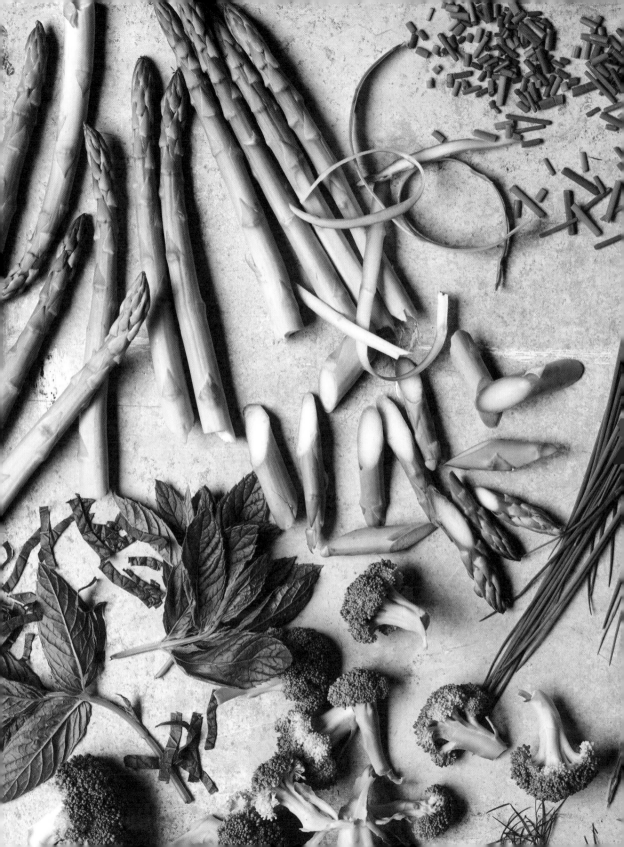

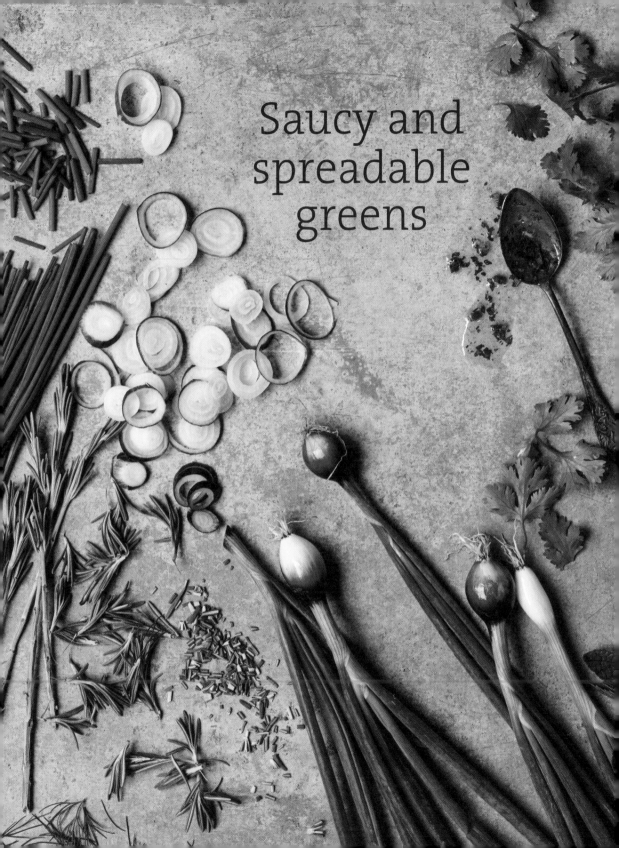

Saucy and
spreadable
greens

Green hummus

I am not a huge fan of canned beans, as they are too squishy and have not been soaked before cooking, which means they are likely to be less digestible and the nutrients harder to assimilate. Dishes also often taste better with freshly cooked beans, and many recipes call for the bean cooking liquid, which contains the flavor and the starch from the cooked beans. If you are short of time, use drained canned chickpeas and fresh water to thin instead. This recipe makes enough for two medium-large jars—use one immediately and freeze the other. MAKES ABOUT 2 CUPS (500ML)

3½oz (100g) Tuscan kale, leaves stripped from the stalks

1 large garlic clove, bashed using the side of a large knife, peeled and coarsely chopped

Scant 2 to 2 cups (270 to 280g) cooked chickpeas (¾ cup/120g dried, see page 152)

2 Tbsp lemon juice

1½ to 2 Tbsp tahini

½ heaping tsp cumin seeds, dry-roasted until fragrant, then ground, plus extra to serve

¼ tsp cayenne pepper, plus extra to serve

Large pinch of sea salt

Chickpea cooking liquid or water

Extra-virgin olive oil, to serve

Briefly steam the kale leaves, or cook in a very small amount of water, until just wilted and bright green. Refresh under cold running water until cool, then squeeze out the excess water.

In a food processor, blitz the keale, garlic, and cooked chickpeas until finely chopped. Add the lemon juice, tahini, cumin, cayenne, and salt and, with the motor running, enough chickpea cooking liquid or water for the hummus to come together, stopping to scrape down the sides as necessary.

If you like a particularly smooth hummus, transfer it to a strong blender and blend until creamy.

Adjust the seasoning and serve with a drizzle of good-quality olive oil, cayenne pepper, and a little ground cumin.

Green butter

This butter is as versatile as it gets—delicious on boiled or baked potatoes, stirred through hot rice or couscous, on toast with egg dishes, with steamed greens, green beans, peas, or asparagus, on steak, with boiled or barbecued corn, and on broiled fish. Freeze it in portions to use as and when the desire strikes. MAKES 1 SMALL LOG—APPROX. 10 TO 15 SLICES

⅔ cup (150g) unsalted butter, cubed and softened

1 Tbsp extra-virgin olive oil

¾ cup (20g/1 small bunch) parsley, leaves only, very finely chopped

½ cup (15g) basil sprigs, leaves only, very finely shredded (see note below)

1 Tbsp finely chopped sage leaves

1 Tbsp finely chopped tarragon leaves

1 large garlic clove, finely chopped

1 Tbsp salted nonpareille (baby) capers, rinsed and finely chopped

Grated zest of 1 lemon

Large pinch of sea salt

Put all the ingredients into a mixing bowl and use an electric whisk to mix well. Alternatively, you could use a food processor, or whisk it all by hand.

Scoop the mixture onto a large rectangular piece of plastic wrap and roll it up like a sausage, spinning the contents around while holding on to the ends, to twist them.

Chill in the refrigerator for at least 4 hours, or until completely firm. Cut off slices to serve as needed, or freeze for later use.

NOTE:
To shred basil, stack the leaves flat on top of each other, then roll into a cigar shape, and slice across into shreds. This method minimizes bruising of the very delicate leaves, as a chopping action turns the edges black.

PHOTOGRAPHED WITH COLLARD GREENS AND PUMPKIN SEED RYE "SOURDOUGH" ON PAGE 138

Parsley pistou

Hardworking parsley is the star of the show in this easy to prepare, yet punchy sauce. Use it in mashed potatoes, with broiled fish, or spread on sandwiches instead of butter. Try adding a drop or two of best-quality orange oil to create something truly uplifting. MAKES ABOUT 250ML

100g (1 large bunch) flat-leaf parsley, leaves only, very finely chopped

1 to 2 garlic cloves, finely chopped

Grated zest of 1–2 oranges

¼ cup (60ml) extra-virgin olive oil

Sea salt and freshly ground black pepper

Mix the parsley, garlic, and orange zest with some salt and black pepper in a small bowl, then slowly add the olive oil in a steady stream, stirring until you've reached the desired consistency. Add a little more oil if you prefer. Season to taste.

If you have an efficient small food processor, you could skip the step of finely chopping the parsley and use the processor to make the pistou instead.

Aji sauce

This spicy, creamy green sauce was made popular by a host of Peruvian restaurants, who serve it with spit-roasted chicken that has first been marinated in olive oil, lime juice, garlic, and spices, then roasted until tender, juicy, and crisp-skinned. You can eat it on almost everything, and it makes a wonderful dip or dressing. I particularly like to use it for potato salads and on boiled eggs. MAKES ENOUGH FOR ROUGHLY 10 TO 12 SERVINGS (ABOUT 1 CUP/250ML)

½ romaine lettuce (about 100g), stem trimmed

1¾oz (50g/1 medium bunch) cilantro, thickest part of stalks removed

5 scallions (about 80g), white and green parts, trimmed and coarsely chopped

2 jalapeño chiles (all or some of the seeds and membranes removed if you want a less spicy version)

1 garlic clove, peeled

Juice of ½ lemon

¼ to ½ cup (60 to 125ml) mayonnaise (see page 154 to make your own, but omit the tarragon)

Sea salt and freshly ground black pepper

Put the lettuce, cilantro, scallions, chiles, garlic, and lemon juice with salt and pepper to taste into a blender and blend until very smooth. You might need to scrape down the sides from time to time to help the blender along.

Pour into a small bowl and whisk in the mayonnaise until the taste and thickness are to your liking. Adjust the seasoning. Store in an airtight container in the refrigerator for up to 1 week.

PHOTOGRAPH ON PAGE 42

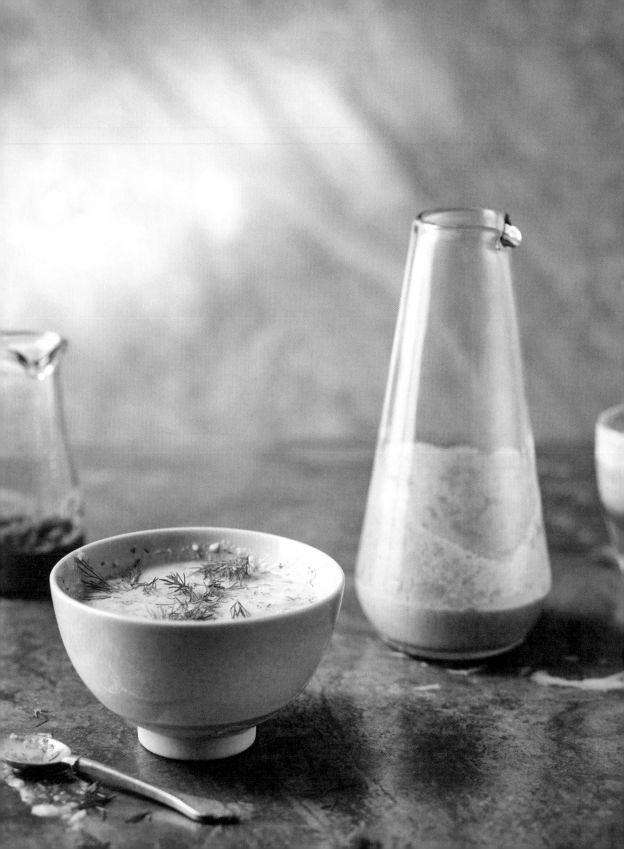

Orange, dill, and fennel dressing

This is ideal for dressing a seafood salad or a celeriac remoulade to accompany broiled fish, but also really delicious as a dressing for crunchy coleslaws or a arugula and roasted beet salad.
MAKES 1 TO 1½ CUPS (250 TO 350ML)

1 whole fennel bulb, outer layer peeled with a vegetable swivel peeler

1½ Tbsp butter or a little oil

¾ cup (180ml) fresh orange juice (2 to 3 oranges)

1 Tbsp cider vinegar

1 Tbsp extra-virgin olive oil

Large pinch of sea salt

1 tsp Dijon mustard

½ tsp anise, dry-roasted and ground (optional)

¾ cup (20g/1 small bunch) dill, tough stems removed, finely chopped

Cut the fennel bulb lengthwise into quarters, then steam in a little water until tender.

Heat the butter in a small pan over medium heat until frothy, then add the cooked fennel, cut sides down. Let caramelize without moving or turning them, until browned around the edges. Remove from the heat and let cool.

Once the fennel has cooled slightly, blend with the orange juice, vinegar, olive oil, salt, mustard, and anise, if using.

Stir in the chopped dill and adjust the seasoning.

Thai dressing

This spicy little number is the perfect dressing for crunchy slaws or noodle salads, or to add some zing to steamed rice, as well as to briefly marinate chicken or fish, and to drizzle over broiled meat. It freezes well.
MAKES ABOUT ½ CUP (125ML)

1 Tbsp coarsely chopped, peeled galangal (or ginger)

1 red chile, trimmed and coarsely chopped (use a Thai chile if you like it very spicy)

2 lemongrass stalks, trimmed, tough outer layers removed, coarsely chopped

1 garlic clove, peeled and bashed with the back of a knife

2 medium scallions, trimmed, green and white parts coarsely chopped

Juice of 2 limes (about 3½ Tbsp)

2 tsp fish sauce

2 tsp tamari or shoyu

2 Tbsp untoasted (virgin) sesame oil or extra-virgin olive oil

1 cup (25g/1 small bunch) cilantro, stems and leaves

2 cups (50g/1 medium bunch) mint, leaves only

1 heaping Tbsp palm sugar (or dark muscovado), or to taste

Put all the ingredients in a blender and blend until smooth.

Left to right: Thai dressing; Orange, dill, and fennel dressing; Aji sauce (recipe on page 41)

Spinach and caramelized onion dip

This is delicious with potato or vegetable chips, tortilla chips, pita chips, or crackers. It could also be stirred through hot pasta or mixed with potato mash. A dollop on the bread roll under burger patties works surprisingly well, and it makes a good omelet when stirred into beaten eggs. Try increasing the amount of cream cheese and filling cannelloni, pasta shells, or ravioli with it. If you leave out the cream cheese to keep it vegan and dairy-free, add a Tbsp or two of olive oil. Finally, you could leave out the cream cheese, not process the ingredients and serve it as a side dish. It freezes well. MAKES ABOUT 1⅔ TO 2 CUPS (400 TO 500ML)

1 Tbsp butter

3 onions (10½ to 12¼oz/300 to 350g), cut in half through the root, then peeled and cut into ¼-in (5-mm) half-moon slices

Large pinch of sea salt

¼ tsp ground cloves

7oz (200g) spinach

1⅓ cups (200g) cooked borlotti beans (see page 152)

1 to 2 Tbsp lemon juice (about 1 small lemon), to taste

¼ cup (50g) light cream cheese, softened

Freshly ground black pepper

Heat the butter in a large saucepan over medium to low heat until just melted, then add the onions, salt, and ground cloves. Cook until soft and translucent, for about 5 minutes, stirring regularly. Do not allow the edges to darken or burn, as this will hinder caramelization.

Turn the heat up to medium and cook for at least 30 minutes, stirring occasionally, until caramelized. If the onions seem to be drying out, stir in a splash of water. Scrape into a food processor.

In the same pan, sauté the spinach until wilted. Let it cool slightly, then squeeze out any excess liquid. Add the spinach and the rest of the ingredients to the food processor with the onions, and process until smooth.

Asparagus and goat curd spread

This is very good as a dip for pita chips or as a filling for crêpes, sandwiches, and omelets served with roasted tomatoes. If you would like to use it as a pasta sauce, set aside the asparagus tips for serving and add a few Tbsp of the pasta cooking liquid to create a saucelike consistency. MAKES ABOUT 1¼ CUPS (300ML)

1 bunch (about 15¾oz/450g) of asparagus spears, trimmed

Olive oil

1 tsp butter

1½ Tbsp shredded sage leaves

2 echalion (banana) shallots, finely diced

1½ to 2 Tbsp lemon thyme leaves, finely chopped

Grated zest of 1 lemon

¼ cup (50g) soft fresh goat curd or rindless soft goat cheese

1 Tbsp lemon juice (about ½ lemon)

Sea salt and freshly ground black pepper

Preheat the oven to 320°F (160°C).

Toss the asparagus in olive oil to coat and season with some salt. Spread out on a lipped baking sheet and roast in the oven for 20 minutes, or until just tender. Set aside to cool.

Meanwhile, heat the butter in a medium saucepan and add the shredded sage leaves. Cook for a few minutes, then increase the heat, add the diced shallots, and cook until they begin to brown around the edges.

Add the chopped thyme and cook for another minute or two, then set aside to cool completely.

Put all the ingredients into a food processor, including the cooled asparagus and shallot mixture, with salt and pepper to taste, and process until smooth. If you want it really smooth, use a blender. Adjust the seasoning and serve or store in a jar in the refrigerator for up to 1 week.

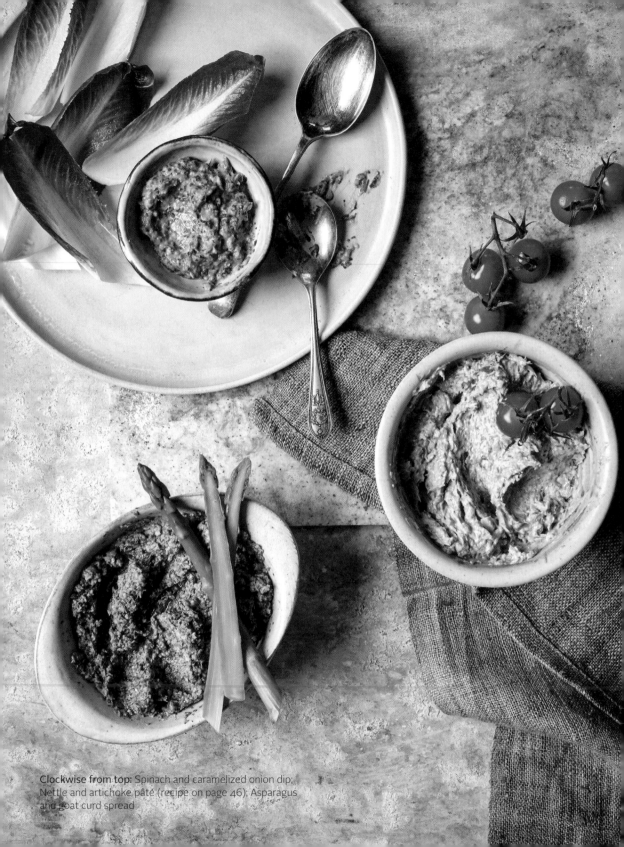

Clockwise from top: Spinach and caramelized onion dip;
Nettle and artichoke pâté (recipe on page 46); Asparagus
and goat curd spread

Nettle and artichoke pâté

Stinging nettles are usually associated with painful encounters, not edible joys. But set aside your prejudices and try this recipe; you will be most surprised! Although the flavor is quite special, nettles can be hard to find, so feel free to use spinach (especially large leaf) instead—just be sure to squeeze out the excess moisture after cooking. If you are a vegan or avoiding dairy, omit the Parmesan and add 1 tsp nutritional yeast flakes. MAKES ABOUT 1 CUP (250ML)

2½ oz (70g) nettle tips (or large-leaf spinach)

1 garlic clove

Large pinch of sea salt

2 to 3 Tbsp lemon juice (1 lemon)

6 oz (170g) drained artichoke hearts in olive oil (about 10oz/280g with the oil)

⅓ cup (50g) pine nuts, toasted until golden

¾ cup (50g) grated Parmesan cheese

Small handful of fresh mint leaves, finely shredded

¼ cup (60ml) extra-virgin olive oil

Freshly ground black pepper

Bring a pan of water to a boil. Wearing gloves, transfer the nettle tips to the boiling water and blanch very briefly until wilted. Drain and let cool, then squeeze out the water and roughly chop.

With a mortar and pestle, grind the garlic clove with the salt until you have a paste.

Add all the ingredients except the olive oil to a food processor and process until smooth. With the motor running, pour in the olive oil in a thin and steady stream until well incorporated.

The end result yields a firm, spreadable pâté. If you would like something a little looser, to stir through pasta or use as a dip for chips, add a Tbsp or two of water and mix again. When cooking pasta, set aside some of the cooking liquid to thin down the sauce.

PHOTOGRAPH ON PAGE 45

Four-herb pesto

This is a vegan version of the popular sauce known and loved in many different cultures. I keep a jar of it in my refrigerator at all times, and if any meal lacks flavor, chlorophyll, or a hit of freshness, this is my trusty go-to. Spread on rye bread, serve with broiled fish, combine with a little yogurt to make a dressing, mix into rice and lentil salads, or mash with avocado for an alternative to guacamole. MAKES 2 CUPS (500ML)

3½ oz (100g/1 large bunch) fresh flat-leaf parsley

3½ oz (100g/1 large bunch) fresh cilantro

7 oz (200g/2 large bunches) fresh basil

2¼ oz (60g) fresh dill sprigs

1 fat garlic clove, peeled

¼ cup (40g) shelled, unroasted macadamia nuts, soaked for a couple of hours, then rinsed

¼ cup (40g) shelled, unroasted pistachios, soaked for a couple of hours, then rinsed

⅓ cup (40g) pine nuts, lightly toasted

½ to 1 cup (125 to 250ml) extra-virgin olive oil

Juice of 1 lemon

Sea salt and freshly ground black pepper

Wash all the herbs and remove the toughest stalks. Dry them separately in a salad spinner, or use a clean dishtowel to bundle up a small bunch of herbs at a time and spin it around.

Put the parsley and garlic into a food processor, and process, then add each of the remaining herbs in order (cilantro, basil, then dill), processing between each addition. Add all the nuts and some salt and pepper, and process.

With the motor running, add enough olive oil in a thin, but steady, stream until the mixture reaches the desired consistency.

Stir in the lemon juice, adjust the seasoning (it needs a fair amount of salt and pepper), and transfer to clean jars. Pour a thin layer of olive oil over the surface of each to seal, put the lids on and store in the refrigerator. Covered in oil, it will keep for several weeks. Alternatively, freeze.

Arugula and almond green sauce

This pungent sauce with a complex flavor is good stirred through pasta, spooned onto broiled fish or chicken, or used to dress a summery peach and mozzarella salad. Use less oil to make a spread that is perfect on pizza bases, or for sandwiches with soft fresh cheese and tomato. You could also stir some Greek yogurt through it to make a salad dressing.
MAKES ABOUT 1 CUP (250ML)

2 medium, hard-boiled egg yolks

About ½ cup (125ml) extra-virgin olive oil

2¼ oz (60g/1 bunch) wild or regular arugula

1¾ oz (50g/1 medium bunch) parsley

Small handful of fresh mint leaves

1 oz (25g/1 bunch) chives

1 large garlic clove, chopped

½ cup (60g) shelled, unsalted almonds, roasted in a 320°F (160°C) oven for about 10 minutes

1 tsp dried red pepper flakes, or to taste (optional)

1 to 2 tsp cider vinegar (or other light vinegar)

Sea salt and freshly ground black pepper

Mash the egg yolks with 1 tsp of the olive oil until you have a smooth paste. Set aside.

Wash the arugula and the herbs, discarding the toughest stalks from the arugula and parsley, and dry separately in a salad spinner or a dishtowel.

Put the arugula and parsley into a food processor and process, then add the mint, chives, garlic, and almonds, and process again. When relatively smooth, add the red pepper flakes, if using, egg yolk paste, vinegar, a very larch pinch of salt, and some pepper, and process for a few more seconds.

With the motor running, add the rest of the oil in a thin, steady stream until it reaches the desired consistency. You may need more, depending on your preferred consistency and how you plan to use it.

Transfer to a clean jar, pour a thin layer of olive oil over the top to seal, put the lid on, and store in the refrigerator for up to 2 weeks. Alternatively, freeze.

Chimichurri

Chimichurri, originally from Argentina, is a very popular green sauce served with all kinds of broiled meats. It is quite simply delicious, and most people—once they have tasted it—admit to eating it on everything, not just meats. The acid in the sauce will turn the herbs a faded green after a couple of days, so eat is as soon as possible after making it and freeze any leftovers. The herbs are traditionally chopped by hand, which can seem quite tedious, but does ensure a lovely texture. If you are pressed for time, though, use a food processor. MAKES 1¼ TO 1½ CUPS (300 TO 350ML)

4 medium garlic cloves

Pinch of rock salt

3¾ cups (100g/1 large bunch) flat-leaf parsley, leaves only, finely chopped

2 cups (50g/1 medium bunch) cilantro, thickest stalks removed, finely chopped

2 Tbsp finely chopped oregano leaves (or 2 tsp dried)

2 Tbsp red wine vinegar

2 Tbsp lemon juice (½ to 1 lemon)

1 red chile, finely chopped (remove seeds and membranes for a milder version) or ½ tsp dried red pepper flakes

1 Tbsp finely chopped shallot (about ½ medium echalion/banana shallot)

Large pinch of sea salt

¾ to 1 cup (180 to 250ml) mild extra-virgin olive oil

Peel the garlic and grind to a paste with the rock salt, using a mortar and pestle. Transfer to a bowl, add the remaining ingredients, except the olive oil, and mix together.

Slowly pour in the oil in a thin, steady stream while stirring, until it reaches the desired consistency.

PHOTOGRAPH ON PAGE 48

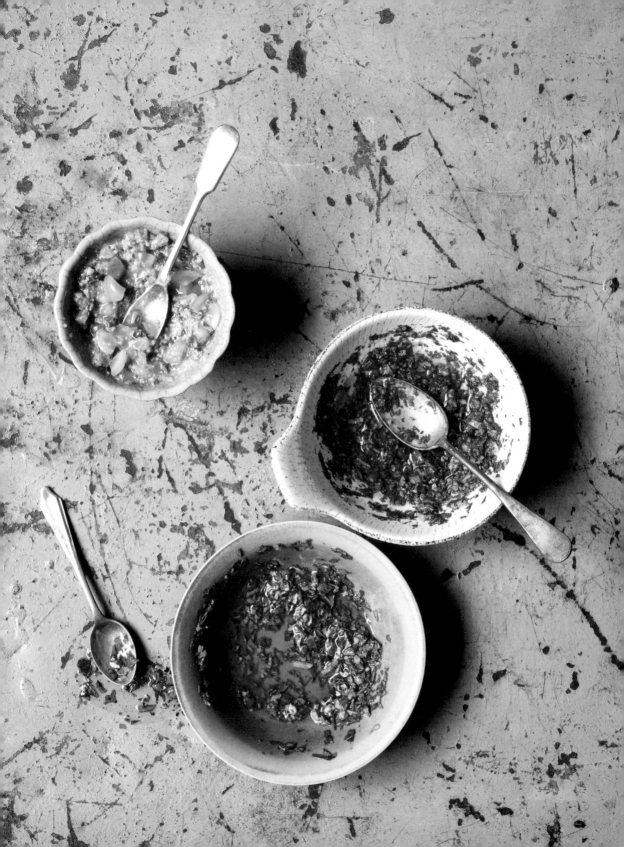

Salsa verde

A timeless classic, salsa verde is delicious with almost everything, but feel free to add a handful of chopped mint leaves and some finely chopped rosemary and replace the lemon juice with red wine vinegar when serving it with lamb. A tsp of Dijon mustard also works well, and 1 Tbsp of chopped tarragon is good when serving it with chicken. Salsa verde is best when the herbs are finely chopped by hand, so resist using a food processor. MAKES ABOUT 1 CUP (250ML)

1oz (25g/1 small bunch) basil, leaves only

2 cups (50g/1 medium bunch) flat-leaf parsley, leaves only, very finely chopped

1 large or 2 small garlic cloves, finely chopped

2 Tbsp capers, rinsed and chopped

5 anchovy fillets in olive oil, mashed with a fork

About ½ cup (125ml) extra-virgin olive oil

3 Tbsp lemon juice (about 1 lemon)

Sea salt and freshly ground black pepper

Working in batches, shred the basil leaves—see Note on page 40 for the best method.

Put the herbs, garlic, capers, and anchovies into a bowl and mix well. Add the olive oil slowly, until it reaches desired consistency. Add the lemon juice with salt and pepper to taste, bearing in mind the anchovies are salty already.

Salsa d'agresto

The word agresto in this traditional sauce from Italy means verjuice (juice from unripe grapes), but I have added green grapes and a couple of anchovies instead to create a delicious, moreish sauce. In Italy it is served with broiled meat and fish, and I eat it on almost everything from roast chicken and pan-fried fish, to crostini with cream cheese or ricotta ravioli. MAKES 1 CUP (250ML)

½ cup (50g) shelled, unroasted walnuts

⅓ cup (50g) shelled, unroasted pecans

2 anchovy fillets in olive oil

1 garlic clove, peeled

1 to generous 1 cup (25 to 30g/1 small bunch) flat-leaf parsley, leaves only, finely chopped

Grated zest and juice of 1 lemon

Pinch of sea salt, or to taste (the anchovies are quite salty)

Freshly ground black pepper, to taste

1⅓ cups (200g) seedless green grapes, washed and finely chopped

½ cup (125ml) extra-virgin olive oil

Taste the walnuts: if they are slightly bitter, use only pecans, or soak them in water for a couple of hours, drain and rinse before using.

Depending on the size of your mortar or suribachi, pound about a third or half of the nuts gently until they start to break up. Add the rest of the nuts and repeat. You should end up with a very grainy texture. Do not overgrind.

Add the anchovies and garlic and continue to pound with the pestle until you have a chunky consistency similar to wet, coarse sand.

Transfer the mixture to a bowl and stir in the rest of the ingredients, except the olive oil. Finally, while stirring continuously, incorporate the olive oil in a thin, steady stream. Adjust the seasoning. Store in an airtight container in the refrigerator for 1 week.

Clockwise from top: Salsa d'agresto; Chimichurri (see recipe on page 47); Salsa verde

Roasted broccoli dip

Consider regularly offering crudités with a dip such as this one at the start of a meal. Research shows that most hungry kids (big and small!) happily snack on these, dramatically increasing their vegetable intake, and even go on to eat more vegetables during the meal. A win-win situation, if you ask me. You could keep this dip dairy-free by replacing the yogurt with natural coconut or nut-based yogurt, available at most healthfood stores. MAKES ABOUT 2 CUPS (500ML)

Preheat the oven to 320°F (160°C).

Rub both cut halves of the garlic bulb with olive oil. Sprinkle with salt and pepper, then place the cut sides back together and wrap in foil.

Wash the broccoli, then separate into florets and dry thoroughly with a clean dishtowel. Toss the florets in some olive oil, salt, and pepper and transfer to a baking sheet, spreading them out in a single layer.

Roast the broccoli and garlic in the oven for 20 to 30 minutes until the broccoli is just cooked through and not burned. Roast the garlic at the same temperature, but for 45 to 60 minutes, until the cloves are soft enough to squeeze from their skins.

Put the remaining ingredients, with salt and pepper to taste, into a food processor or blender and add the roasted broccoli and squeezed out garlic. Process until smooth, scraping down the sides a few times if necessary.

If you like your dip a little runnier, add small amounts of hot water with the motor running, or more yogurt.

PHOTOGRAPHED HERE WITH NORI AMARANTH CRACKERS
(RECIPE ON PAGE 136)

1 whole unpeeled garlic bulb, cut in half horizontally

¼ cup (60ml) extra-virgin olive oil, plus extra for the garlic and broccoli

1 small head of broccoli

Generous 1 cup (175g) cooked light-colored beans, such as lima beans or cannellini (see page 152)

1 oz (25g/1 small bunch) parsley

1 oz (25g/1 small bunch) cilantro

¼ cup (60ml) goat or cow yogurt

Sea salt and freshly ground black pepper

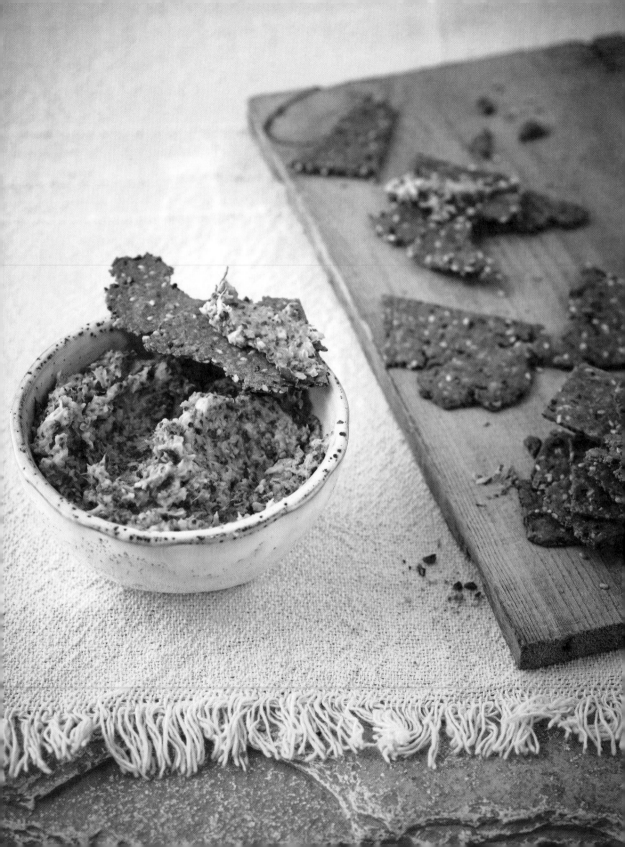

Smoked mackerel and watercress mousse

Serve this as an indulgent appetizer on Watercress Oat Cakes (page 136), or as first course or light lunch with wafer-thin toasted sourdough and the Sea Vegetable Salad (page 119).
MAKES 1½ CUPS (375ML)

Using plastic wrap, line a mini loaf pan or a mold that will hold 1½ cups (375ml) liquid, making sure the plastic wrap hangs over the sides (to help unmold the mousse).

Blitz the watercress in a food processor until fine, then add the smoked mackerel and pulse a few times until coarsely chopped. Transfer to a bowl and stir in the sour cream and horseradish sauce. Season with a little salt and plenty of pepper, and set aside.

If using powdered gelatin, whisk the granules into the broth and wine in a small saucepan and let soften for 1 minute. Gently heat over low heat until all the granules have dissolved. Set aside to cool slightly before stirring into the fish and cream mixture.

If using leaf gelatin, submerge the leaves in a bowl of room temperature water and let soften for 4 to 5 minutes. Meanwhile, gently heat the broth and wine in a small pan over low heat. Drain the softened gelatin sheets, squeeze out the excess water, add to the warm liquid, and whisk until fully dissolved. Set aside to cool slightly before stirring into the fish and cream mixture.

If using agar agar, slowly bring the broth and wine to a boil in a pan with the agar agar, whisking continuously. If you heat it too rapidly, the agar will form little beads of hard gel. Once the flakes have completely dissolved, remove from the heat and let cool only slightly before stirring into the fish mixture.

Adjust the seasoning, bearing in mind that jelling and refrigeration tend to tone flavors down. Scrape the mixture into the prepared mold, then refrigerate until firm, for at least 4 hours. When the mousse has set, lift it out of the mold with the help of the plastic wrap. Place a serving plate face down on the mousse, then flip both over and remove the plastic wrap. Serve with lemon wedges and a few watercress sprigs.

PHOTOGRAPHED HERE WITH WATERCRESS OAT CAKES (RECIPE ON PAGE 136) AND SEA VEGETABLE SALAD (RECIPE ON PAGE 119)

1¾ oz (50g) watercress, stalks and leaves, plus a few sprigs to garnish

3½ oz (100g) smoked mackerel

¼ cup (60ml) sour cream

¼ cup (60ml) horseradish sauce (or see page 156 to make your own)

Enough powdered or leaf gelatin to set 1 cup (250ml) liquid (about 1½ tsp powdered or 3 gelatin leaves), or 1½ Tbsp agar agar flakes

⅓ cup (80ml) fish or vegetable broth

¼ cup (60ml) white wine (or more broth)

Sea salt and freshly ground black pepper

Lemon wedges, to serve

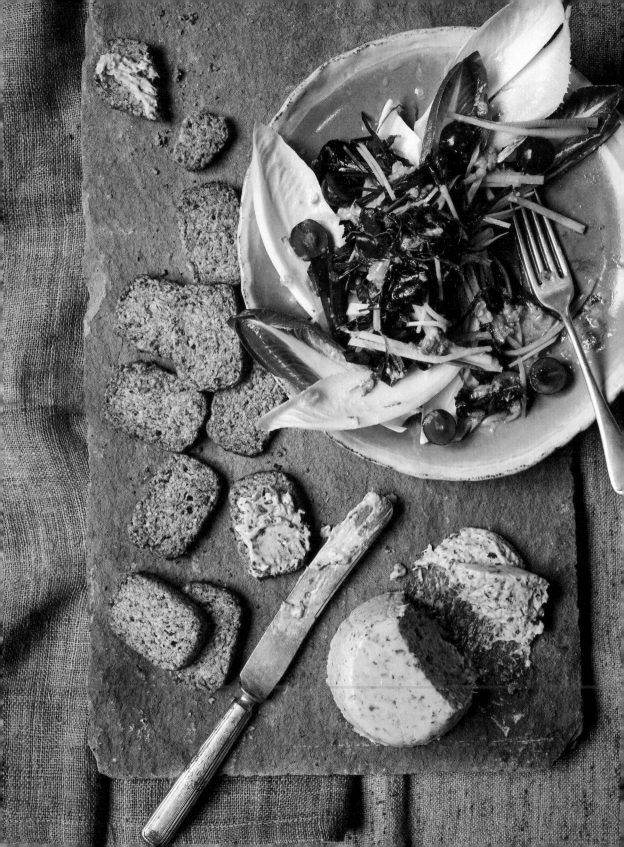

Fresh chive ricotta

If you've never had freshly made ricotta, you're in for a treat. The beauty of it is its simplicity and subtle taste, and with vibrant green chive oil, it becomes super versatile. Either mix some oil into the ricotta and use as a topping on crostini or in pasta dishes; or set aside the oil to drizzle over ricotta pancakes or soups. It has to be prepared a day ahead to give the chives a chance to flavor the oil, but it is little effort. The leftover whey from the ricotta can be used in place of water in baking recipes or in smoothies. MAKES 1LB 2OZ (500G) RICOTTA AND ½ CUP (125ML) CHIVE OIL

For the chive oil, bring a small pan of water to a boil and blanch the chives for 20 seconds, then drain and refresh under cold running water, or tip into a bowl of iced water.

Wrap the chives up in a dishtowel and swing it around to shake off any excess water, then blend with the oil until the chives have been completely incorporated. Pour into a glass jar, put the lid on, and infuse in the refrigerator for 24 hours. Strain the oil through a nut milk bag or a few layers of cheesecloth to remove any pulp.

To make the ricotta, line a colander with a double layer of cheesecloth and set it over a large bowl. Pour the milk into a large, heavy-bottom pan that is wider than it is high, and heat gradually over medium heat until almost boiling. The milk should be foamy and starting to steam and bubble around the edges. If a skin has formed, scoop it off and discard.

Reduce the heat to low and add the lemon juice or vinegar and the salt. Stir gently once or twice to distribute the acid, but don't stir more than twice, as it could result in chewy curds. Leave the milk undisturbed for 10 minutes, after which it should have separated into clumps of milky white curds and thin, watery, yellow whey. Dip a slotted spoon in to check; if you still see a lot of unseparated milk, add another Tbsp of lemon juice or vinegar and wait a few more minutes.

Using a slotted spoon, carefully scoop the big curds out of the pan and into the lined colander. Pour any remaining small curds and the whey through the colander, being careful not to break up the larger ones. Let the curds drain for 5 to 10 minutes, depending on how moist you like your cheese.

Scoop the ricotta into a bowl and whisk in the lemon zest and generous amounts of black pepper, with more salt if it needs it. You can store it in an airtight container in the refrigerator for a few days at this stage.

Now, you can choose to add the chive oil directly to the ricotta or set it all aside for drizzling. If adding, do so bit by bit, tasting along the way until you are happy with the balance. I usually incorporate 3 to 4 Tbsp of the oil. Serve immediately, drizzled with more chive oil, a grating of black pepper, some lemon zest, and perhaps a few red pepper flakes or sweet paprika.

FOR THE CHIVE OIL

1 cup (25g/1 bunch) chives, cut into thirds

½ cup (125ml) extra-virgin olive oil

FOR THE RICOTTA

8 cups (2L) whole milk of your choice (cow, goat, or sheep)

¼ cup (60 ml) lemon juice (1½ to 2 lemons) or white wine vinegar

1 tsp salt

Grated zest of 1 large lemon, plus extra to serve

Freshly ground black pepper and coarse sea salt

Dried red pepper flakes or sweet paprika, to serve (optional)

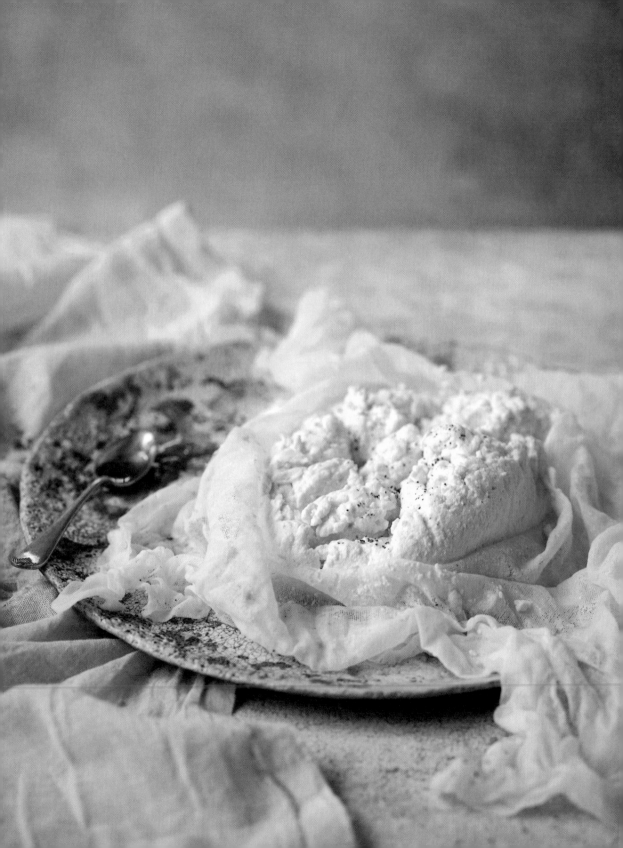

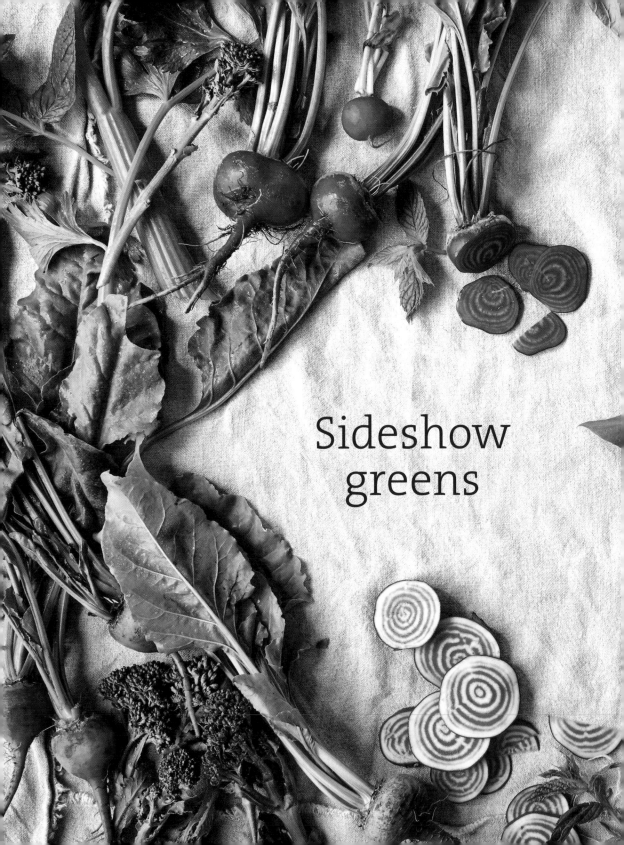

Sideshow greens

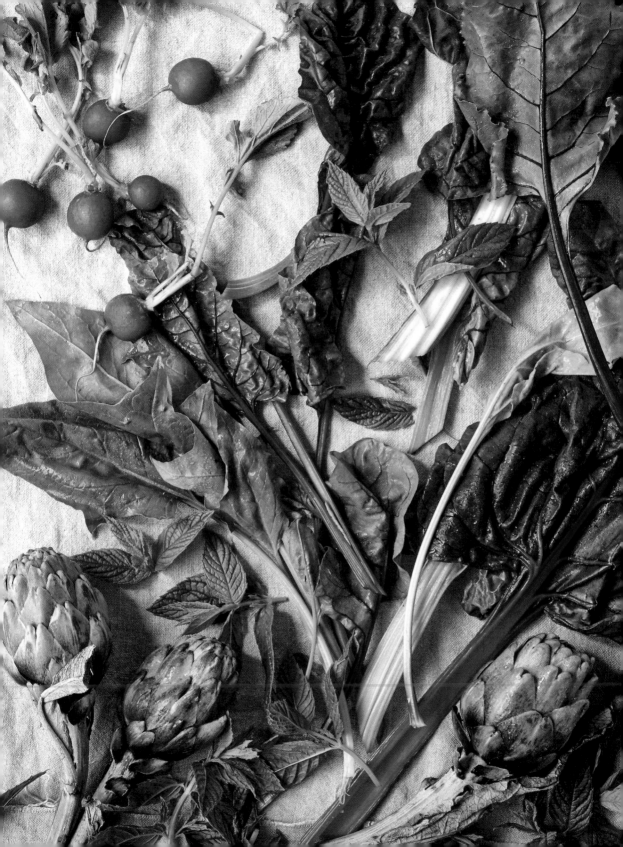

Pumpkin and sprout "truffles" with dukkha

My three-year-old wolfs these down, so I can say with confidence that it is a family-friendly recipe. However, it does take time to prepare and is more of a weekend or festive-occasion dish. Be sure to use pumpkin/squash that has a dry flesh, as this will give you a malleable mixture and not a sloppy mess. The dukkha makes about 2 cups of deliciousness to sprinkle on salads, avocado toasties, or baked bananas, or to use alongside olive oil as a dip for fresh crusty bread. MAKES ABOUT 24

Preheat the oven to 400°F (200°C).

Toss the pumpkin in the oil or ghee and some salt, then spread out on a baking sheet in a single layer and roast for 30 to 50 minutes, turning the pieces once, until caramelized and dry roasted. If the pumpkin looks as though it is still steaming (or sweating), roast for another 5 to 10 minutes. Let cool completely before mashing until smooth, then transfer to a bowl.

While the pumpkin is baking, spread the hazelnuts out on a baking sheet and roast for 10 to 15 minutes. Rub between two clean dishtowels to remove the skins, then let cool.

Finely chop the cooled hazelnuts in the small bowl of a food processor, until there are no large pieces but they still retain lots of texture. Alternatively, use a sharp knife. Mix with all the other dukkha ingredients in a bowl and set aside.

Heat a little oil or ghee in a saucepan and fry the caraway seeds until fragrant. Add the sprouts and cook, stirring regularly, until tender. Tip out onto a cutting board and use a large knife to chop up finely. Mix with the cranberries in the bowl of mashed pumpkin and season generously with salt.

Using a teaspoon, scoop small amounts of pumpkin mixture into your hand and roll into balls. If the mixture still feels too moist to roll into truffles, add a few spoonfuls of quinoa or fine oat flakes until the mixture becomes manageable.

Working in batches, pour some dukkha into a soup bowl and roll the truffles in the dukkha until well covered. Continue until all the truffles are coated, then serve.

FOR THE TRUFFLES

1 medium (about 2¼lb/1kg) dry-fleshed pumpkin or squash (such as onion squash), peeled, seeded, and cut into medium dice

½ Tbsp grapeseed oil, or melted coconut oil or ghee, plus extra for frying

½ tsp caraway seeds

4¼oz (120g) Brussels sprouts, trimmed, halved, and very thinly sliced

⅓ cup (40g) dried cranberries, coarsely chopped

Sea salt

FOR THE DUKKHA

1 cup (125g) shelled, unroasted hazelnuts

1 Tbsp cumin seeds, toasted in a dry frying pan until fragrant

1 Tbsp ground coriander

⅓ cup (50g) sesame seeds, toasted in a dry frying pan until golden

1 heaping Tbsp dried mint (or use the contents of a mint teabag)

2 tsp nigella seeds

1 tsp sea salt

½ tsp freshly ground black pepper (or less if feeding children)

2 tsp dulse flakes (optional)

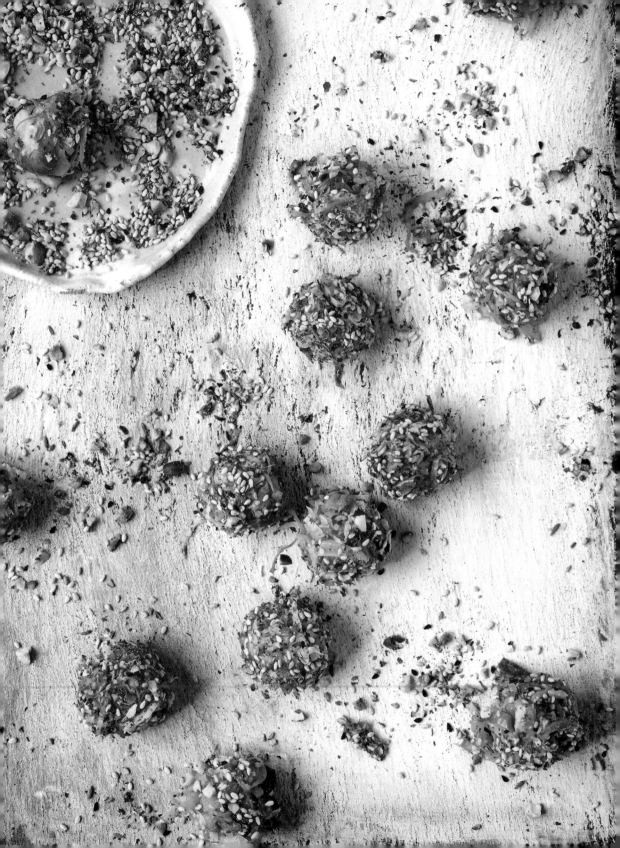

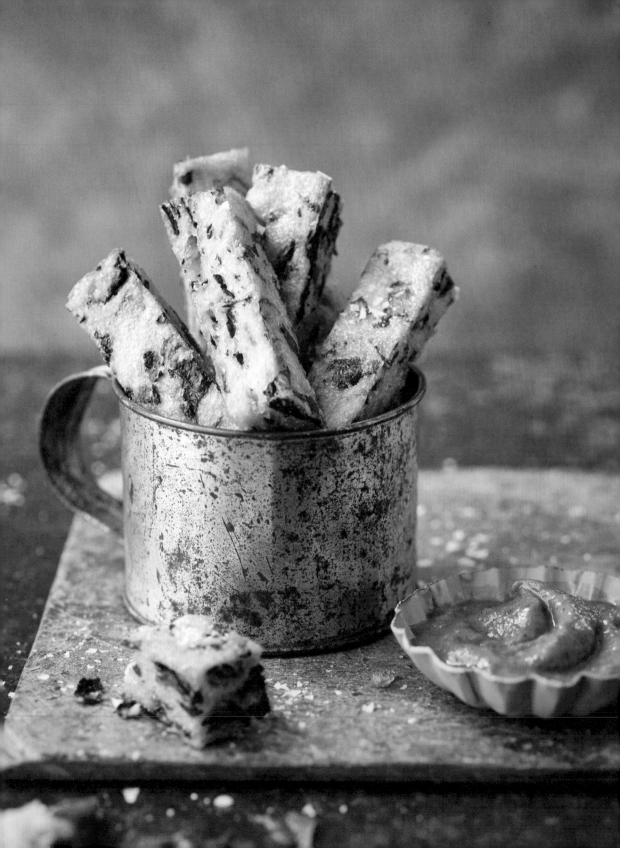

Polenta and Swiss chard chips with rich tomato sauce

This is usually a hit with kids and very easy to make, but requires a little planning ahead. The polenta needs to be made and then cooled completely before being cut and roasted. If you can't find chard, use any dark leafy green of your choice. SERVES 4 TO 6

Cut the stalks off the chard leaves, chop them into small pieces, and set aside. Chop the leaves into bite-size pieces and set aside, separately.

Melt the butter in a large, deep saucepan, add the onion with a pinch of salt, and sweat over medium heat. Add the chard stalks and sauté for 5 to 10 minutes until tender, then add the leaves and sauté for a minute longer.

Add the boiling water to the pan and stir in the cornmeal. Whisk until thickened, then stir in 1 tsp salt and some pepper, cover, and cook over low heat for 10 to 20 minutes. Pour into an ovenproof dish and flatten with the back of a metal spoon to an even thickness of about 1¼in (3cm) or, if your dish is large enough, ⅝in (1.5cm). Let set and ideally refrigerate for a few hours.

Preheat the oven to 400°F (200°C).

When the polenta is completely firm, cut into "chips" about ⅝ by ⅝in (1.5 by 1.5cm) thick and 3in (8cm) long. Place all the chips on a baking sheet close together and brush on all sides with melted coconut oil, ghee, or grapeseed oil.

Spread the chips out a little and roast in the oven for about 1 hour, until golden and crunchy on the outside, carefully turning them with a spatula after 30 minutes. Serve hot with the warmed Rich Tomato Sauce.

7 oz (200g) Swiss or rainbow chard, washed well

A little butter

1 medium onion, peeled and finely diced

5½ cups (1.3L) boiling water

2 cups (280g) medium or coarse cornmeal

Melted coconut oil or ghee, or grapeseed oil, for brushing

Sea salt and freshly ground black pepper

¼ quantity of Rich Tomato Sauce (page 153), warmed, to serve

Savory oatmeal
with Asian greens

If you are in need of a side dish that stands its ground, this is the one. It is earthy and comforting, yet fragrant and cheeky. It sits nicely alongside good pastured meat or line-caught fish, though for me a poached or fried egg is the most perfect partner of all. SERVES 4 GENEROUSLY

For the oatmeal, put the oats, galangal, salt, and lemongrass in a medium saucepan. Add the hot water or broth and the coconut milk. Bring to a boil, then reduce the heat to low and simmer for 30 to 35 minutes, stirring frequently.

Five minutes before the oatmeal is ready, for the Asian greens, heat the coconut oil in a wok or large frying pan. When the oil is hot, but before it reaches smoking point, add the scallions and chiles, cook for 1 minute, then add the garlic and ginger, cooking for another minute while stirring continuously.

Add the snow peas and stir-fry for a minute before adding the greens and salt. Once the greens have wilted, add the broccoli and Thai basil and stir until the basil has wilted. Serve immediately on top of the oatmeal.

FOR THE OATMEAL

2½ cups (240g) pinhead oats

A few slices of fresh or dried galangal (or ginger)

1 tsp sea salt

1 lemongrass stalk, cut into thirds and bashed with the back of a knife

2 cups (480ml) hot water, vegetable broth, or fresh chicken broth

2½ cups (600ml) coconut milk (about 1½ cans)

FOR THE ASIAN GREENS

1 Tbsp coconut oil

4 scallions, white and green part, trimmed and diagonally sliced

1 to 2 red chiles, sliced (seeds and membranes removed if you prefer less heat)

2 garlic cloves, finely chopped

1 Tbsp grated peeled ginger

7oz (200g) snow peas, trimmed and any strings removed

1 small bunch (about 10½oz/300g) of collard greens, thick cores discarded and leaves roughly chopped

1 tsp sea salt

7oz (200g) purple sprouting, tenderstem, or regular broccoli, briefly steamed and refreshed under cold water

1oz (25g/1 small bunch) Thai basil (or regular basil), leaves only

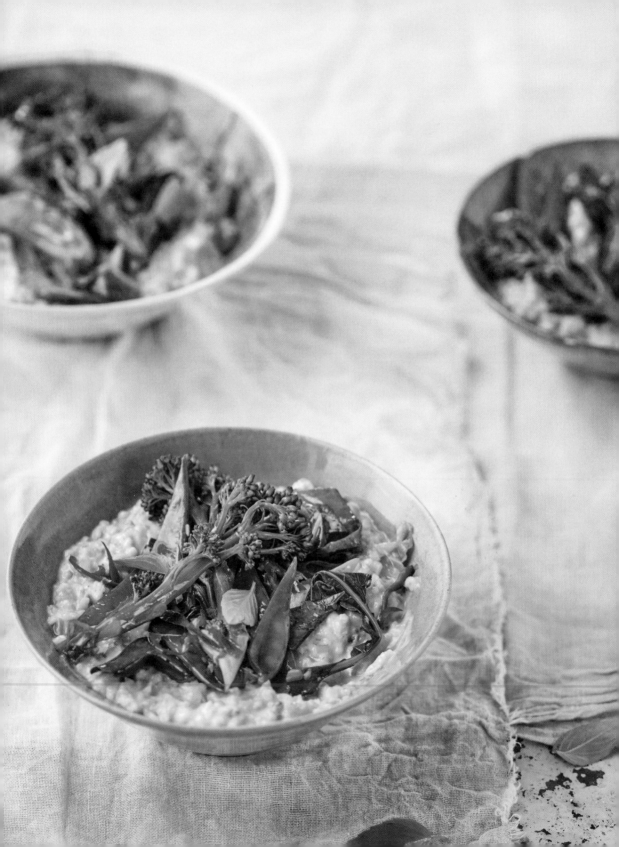

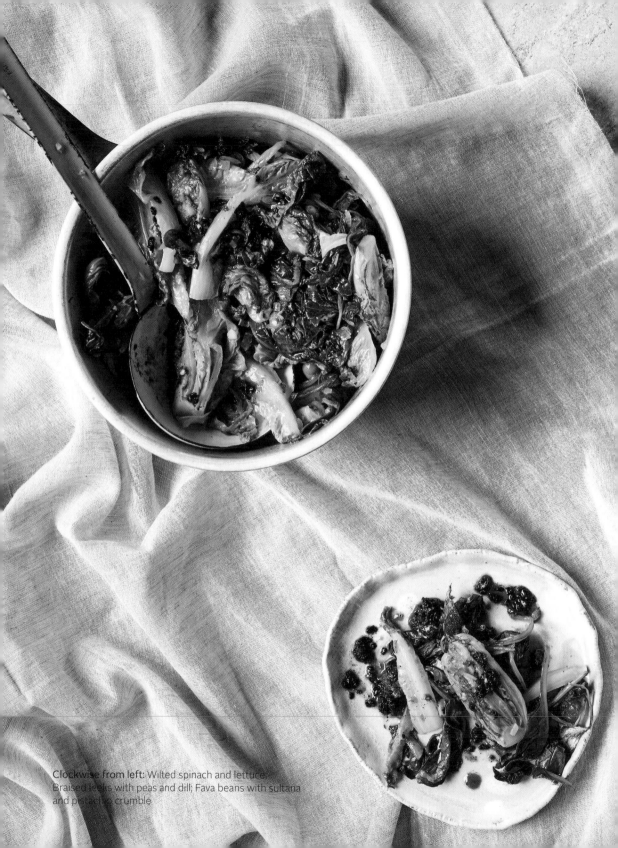

Clockwise from left: Wilted spinach and lettuce;
Braised leeks with peas and dill; Fava beans with sultana
and pistachio crumble

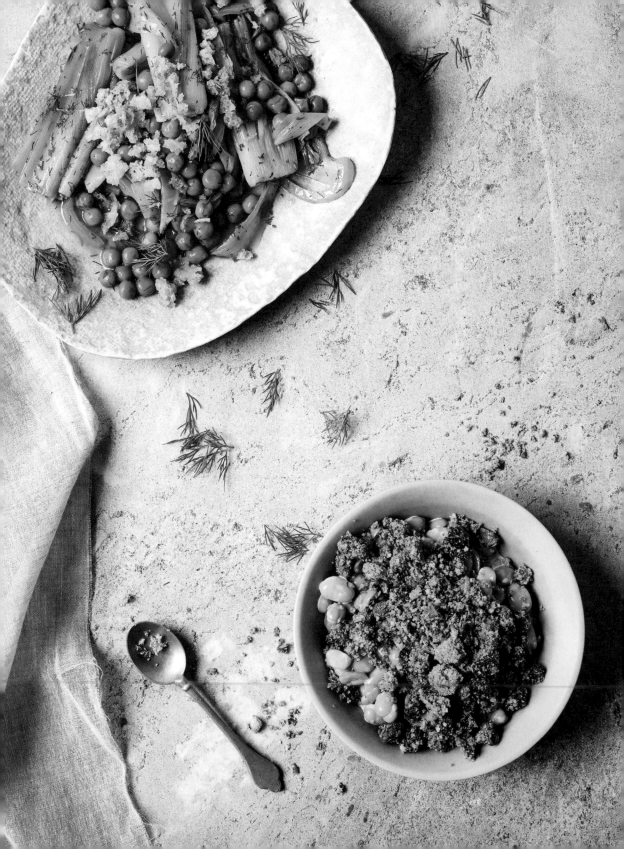

Fava beans with golden raisin and pistachio crumble

This is a family favorite and you will see why once you've tasted it. To double-pod fresh, mature fava beans, remove the beans from the outer pods, then boil them for a couple of minutes and shock under cold water. Next, slip off the gray, leathery skins to reveal the luminous green bean inside. Simply blanch frozen fava beans very briefly in boiling water. SERVES 4 TO 5

10½oz (300g) fresh (or 11¼oz/320g frozen) double-podded fava beans (from approx. 2½lb/1.2kg beans in their pods)

A few Tbsp of Tarragon Mayonnaise (page 154)

FOR THE CRUMBLE
Generous ⅓ cup (50g) wholewheat spelt flour or gluten-free flour mix

3½ Tbsp cold butter or cold coconut butter, cut into small cubes

¼ cup (25g) quinoa flakes or fine oat flakes

Pinch of sea salt

⅓ cup (50g) shelled, unroasted pistachios

¼ cup (50g) golden raisins

Preheat the oven to 350°F (180°C).

Put the spelt flour, cold butter, quinoa flakes, and salt in a food processor and pulse until it starts to come together. Now add the pistachios and golden raisins, and pulse a few more times. Scrape into a bowl and knead a little to form a dough.

Break the dough into large chunks (your aim is crunchy nuggets of crumble the size of granola clusters) onto a lipped baking sheet and bake for 20 to 30 minutes or until the crumble is golden and crispy. Remove and let cool.

A few minutes before the crumble is ready, steam the fava beans very briefly to heat. Mix with 2 to 3 Tbsp Tarragon Mayonnaise and arrange on a plate. Sprinkle the toasted crumble over and serve immediately as it does not keep very well.

FIRST THREE DISHES PHOTOGRAPHED ON PAGES 64 TO 65

Braised leeks with peas and dill

This is the kind of dish that feels luxurious, although it is easy to make and not at all exotic. SERVES 4 TO 5

1 Tbsp butter

1 Tbsp extra-virgin olive oil, plus extra to drizzle

1lb 2oz (500g) trimmed leeks, halved lengthwise, then cut into 4-in (10-cm) pieces

Large pinch of sea salt

1 large fennel bulb, outer layer peeled with a vegetable swivel peeler, halved lengthwise, and sliced

1 cup (250ml) hot vegetable broth

½ cup (125ml) dry sherry (or extra broth)

½ tsp ground anise

2 large, thick slices sourdough bread, cut into chunks

1 cup (150g) fresh or frozen peas

⅓ cup (10g/½ small bunch) dill, larger stalks removed, finely chopped

Sea salt and freshly ground black pepper

Preheat the oven to 320°F (160°C).

Heat the butter and oil in a large saucepan that will fit the vegetables snugly. Add the leeks, cut sides down, and a large pinch of salt. After a few minutes, turn them over and sauté for another few minutes before adding the fennel, broth, sherry if using, anise, and some black pepper. Cover and braise over low heat for 20 to 30 minutes, or until the leeks and fennel are tender.

Meanwhile, process the bread to coarse crumbs in a food processor, tip onto a lipped baking sheet, sprinkle with salt and pepper and a good drizzle of olive oi, and spread out in a single layer. Bake for 20 to 25 minutes or until golden and crunchy.

Using a slotted spoon, transfer the cooked vegetables to a bowl, leaving the sauce in the pan, and keep warm. Simmer the sauce over high heat for 5 to 10 minutes until reduced by three-quarters. Stir in the peas and, as soon as they are warm, add the dill. Return the vegetables to the pan and mix.

Top with the crispy sourdough crumbs and serve immediately as it does not keep very well.

Wilted spinach and lettuce

This is one of my favorite recipes in this book, and the type of dish that my kids happily eat if I chop it up finely. The black sesame seeds can be a pain to find if you don't have a good local ethnic grocer near you, but you can use hulled white ones instead. SERVES 2 TO 4

Grapeseed oil or melted coconut oil

1 large shallot, finely chopped

2 Boston lettuces, trimmed, leaving the core intact, rinsed, and quartered lengthwise

1 large or 2 small garlic cloves, finely chopped

7 to 8¾oz (200 to 250g) baby leaf spinach

FOR THE DRESSING
1 tsp traditionally fermented organic soy sauce, tamari, or shoyu (see Note on page 88)

1 tsp umeboshi vinegar (also called umeboshi seasoning) or brown rice vinegar

1 tsp untoasted (virgin) sesame oil

1 Tbsp white and black sesame seeds, lightly toasted in a dry frying pan until white ones are golden

½ tsp honey

Pinch of kombu (kelp) flakes (optional)

½ tsp ground Szechuan pepper

1 tsp freshly ground nutmeg

Grated zest of 1 tangerine

Make the dressing by combining all the ingredients in a jar and shaking to dissolve the honey.

Heat some oil in a large pan and cook the shallot until soft and translucent. Scrape to the edges of the pan, increase the heat a tad, and place the lettuce quarters, cut sides down, in the pan, adding a little more oil if necessary.

When the lettuce pieces have caramelized, turn them over, add the garlic and spinach, and keep moving the spinach around as it starts to wilt.

As soon as all the spinach has wilted, pour over the dressing, toss, adjust the seasoning, and serve immediately as it does not keep very well.

Green beans, artichokes, and olives

Most people love green beans and I usually serve them as a side in some shape or form. This dish is a little more daring than the usual green bean fare, but feel free to omit the olives if you wish. If you are making this in advance, remember that the acid in the lemon juice will turn the lovely bright-green beans an army green after a little while, so dress the beans just before serving. SERVES 4 TO 6

10½oz (300g) fine green beans, trimmed

1 medium garlic clove, finely chopped

1½ Tbsp extra-virgin olive oil (if you can find orange-infused olive oil, even better)

1½ Tbsp lemon juice (about ½ large lemon)

6¼oz (175g) broiled artichokes in oil, drained and quartered if large

½ cup (50g) Spanish Couchillo olives (or any other small black olives)

Grated zest of 1 orange

Sea salt, to taste (the olives are quite salty)

Steam the beans in a little water until just tender. Drain immediately and refresh under cold running water until completely cooled.

Put the beans with the remaining ingredients in a bowl and toss well to mix.

Flower sprouts with anchovies and roasted garlic

Flower sprouts are a newly developed vegetable that look like tiny cabbages with green frilly leaves and streaks of purple. They are related to Brussels sprouts, but have a more subtle flavor and are richer in vitamins B6 and C. In this recipe you could substitute steamed Tuscan kale or other leafy greens for the flower sprouts. SERVES 4

1 Tbsp extra-virgin olive oil

3 anchovy fillets in oil

½ quantity of Roasted Garlic (page 154)

8¾oz (250g) steamed flower sprouts

Lemon juice, to taste

Sea salt and freshly ground black pepper

Gently heat the olive oil in a large pan and add the anchovies and garlic, squeezed out of its skins. Use a fork to mash both into the oil.

Increase the heat a little, shake off any excess liquid from the steamed flower sprouts, and add to the pan. Sauté for a few minutes, add salt and pepper to taste, and squeeze over some lemon juice. Serve immediately.

Broccoli and carrot tabbouleh

This is an easy way to get your kids to eat broccoli and an even easier way to make some very basic ingredients taste rather good. You could easily replace the costly pistachios with a seed or nut of your choice. SERVES 4

Glug of good olive oil

1 small onion, finely diced

1½ to 2 cups (200 to 250g) finely grated carrot (about 2 medium carrots)

10½ oz (300g/1 small head) broccoli, broken into florets

1⅔ cups (300g) cooked quinoa (about 1 cup/ 150g uncooked grain)

Scant ⅓ to ⅔ cup (90 to 100g) shelled, unroasted pistachios

Sea salt

FOR THE DRESSING
5 Tbsp extra-virgin olive oil

Juice of 1 lemon (about 2 Tbsp)

Grated zest of 1 lemon

⅓ cup (10g/½ bunch) chives, finely chopped

1 garlic clove, finely chopped

½ tsp Dijon mustard

1 tsp maple syrup

Heat the glug of oil in a saucepan over gentle heat, add the onion and a pinch of salt, and sweat until soft and translucent. Add the grated carrot and cook for a few more minutes.

Blitz the broccoli in a food processor until fine. Add to the onions and cook for another couple of minutes until both the carrot and the broccoli are tender. Transfer to a serving dish.

Combine all the dressing ingredients with a pinch of salt in a glass jar, screw the lid on tightly, and give it a good shake.

Pour the dressing over the warm vegetables and mix. Add the quinoa and nuts, mix well, and serve. (It is also very good the next day.)

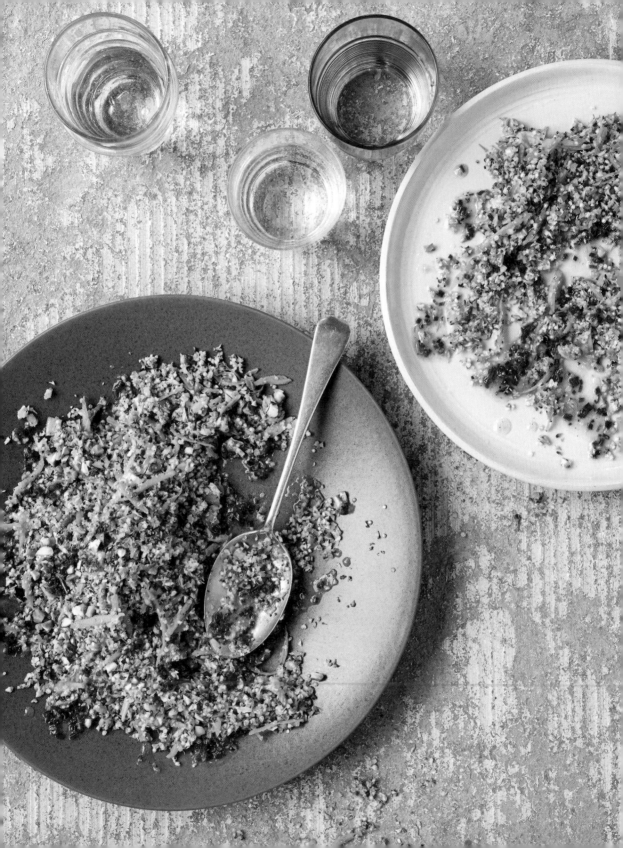

Napa cabbage kimchi

Please trust me when I say that this is simpler than it looks. Kimchi is chock-full of healthy gut-supportive probiotics and really quite delicious, adding spice and pizzazz to almost anything, from roast chicken or fish, to pancakes and polenta. The method of blending the apple with the spices is something I learned from food preservationist extraordinaire, Michaela Hayes of Crock & Jar. I have kept this version vegan, so replaced the traditional fish or shrimp sauce with kelp flakes. But do add some sauce if you like—it is more authentic that way. MAKES 1 MEDIUM TO LARGE JAR, BUT YOU WILL NEED A LARGE JAR FOR FERMENTATION

Cut the cabbage lengthwise into quarters and then across into 4 to 2-in (5-cm) strips. Put into a large bowl with the salt. Massage the salt into the cabbage until it starts to soften (I usually wear kitchen gloves to do this), then add enough cold water, ideally filtered, to cover the cabbage. Put a plate on top, weigh it down with a few cans, and set aside to brine for 2 to 3 hours.

Rinse the cabbage well under cold water to get rid of most of the saltiness and set aside to drain in a colander for 30 minutes.

Meanwhile, process the garlic, ginger, shallots, apple, tamari, kelp flakes, if using, and water in a small food processor or using a stick blender, until you have a smooth paste. Mix in the gochugaru, using 1 Tbsp for a mild version and up to 5 for a spicy end result (I usually use 2½).

Mix the paste into the carrots, scallions, and radishes. Gently squeeze any remaining water from the cabbage and return it to the bowl along with the vegetables and paste. Mix thoroughly with a large spoon or gloved hands.

Pack the kimchi into a large jar that has ample room at the top to avoid any overflow, pressing down firmly on it until the juices rise to cover the vegetables. On the first day, the liquid might not be quite enough to cover all the vegetables, but it should be by day 2 at the latest. Seal the jar with the lid.

Let the jar stand at room temperature for 2 to 5 days, checking and tasting it daily, always pressing the vegetables down under the liquid with a clean spoon. Remember to do this at least once a day, as you don't want the gases to build up and the jar to explode. As soon as you like the taste, transfer to the refrigerator. I prefer my kimchi when it is not overly fermented or "ripe," so usually eat it within a few weeks of transferring it to the refrigerator, but it keeps well for several months if covered in brine and refrigerated.

1 head (1¼lb/600 to 650g) of napa cabbage (you could also use green, white, or savoy cabbage, although the end result will be slightly different)

⅓ cup (65g) unrefined coarse sea salt

6 garlic cloves

⅜-in (1-cm) piece of ginger, peeled and grated

2 shallots (about 1 cup/90g), coarsely chopped

1 apple, cored and coarsely chopped

2 Tbsp tamari

Large pinch of kelp flakes (optional)

2 Tbsp water

1 to 5 Tbsp gochugaru (Korean red pepper flakes), or regular dried red pepper flakes

3 medium carrots (about 10½oz/300g), peeled and cut into matchsticks or thin rounds

5 scallions, green and white parts, trimmed and cut into 5mm slices

5¼oz (150g) radishes, trimmed and halved if large

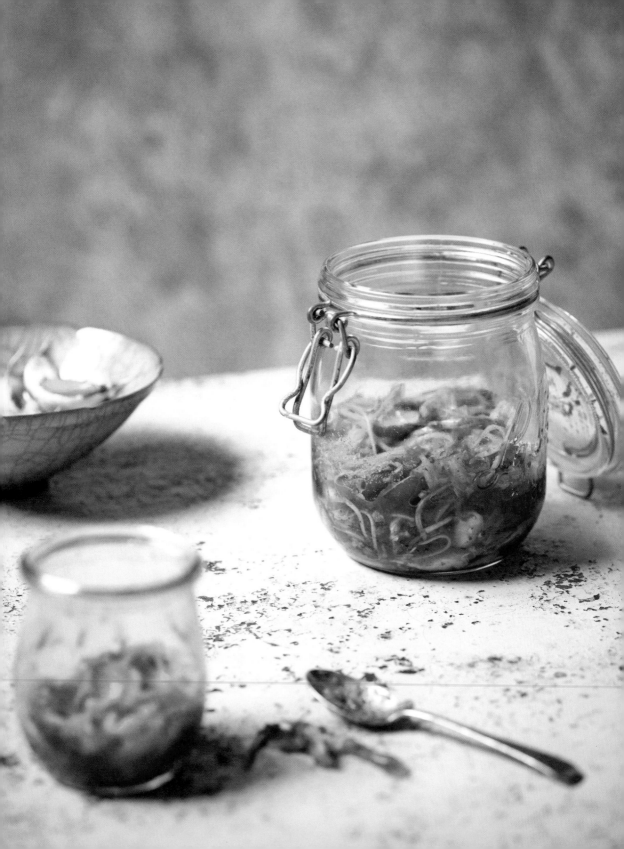

Swiss chard with ginger and tomato sauce

I'll admit this dish is not about the chard. It is about the sauce. Even though the chard (or any wilted leafy green for that matter) tastes great in it, the sauce is also a fantastic overnight marinade for meat, fish, or chicken that is destined for the barbecue. The recipe makes more than enough sauce for the chard, but I usually double or triple it to refrigerate or freeze. And if the leftover candied ginger is causing you anxiety, try stirring it into pancake or chocolate cake batter, mixing it into cookie dough or adding it to Asian-style vinaigrettes. SERVES 2 TO 4

½ cup (125ml) Rich Tomato Sauce (page 153)

½ cup (125ml) passata (strained tomatoes)

1 Tbsp tomato paste

1 Tbsp grated peeled ginger

¼ tsp ground ginger

1 Tbsp (about 15g) finely chopped candied ginger

½ tsp sweet paprika

½ Tbsp dark muscovado sugar

½ Tbsp lemon juice

1½ Tbsp of butter or a little coconut oil

4 cups (300g) Swiss chard, washed, stalks chopped, and leaves cut into bite-size pieces

Sea salt

Put all the ingredients, except the butter and chard, into a small saucepan, add a large pinch of salt, and simmer over low heat for 20 to 30 minutes, stirring regularly to avoid it catching on the bottom.

Just before the sauce is ready, heat the butter or coconut oil in a pan and sauté the chard stalks with a large pinch of salt until tender. Add the leaves and cook until wilted.

Spoon enough sauce over to coat all the chard. Serve with broiled fish and steamed rice, or alongside a light and fluffy savory soufflé.

Watercress, mango, and avocado salsa

Wonderful with pan-fried or broiled fish or roast chicken, and as an accompaniment to roasted corn, broiled halloumi, or toasted sandwiches, this salsa is a grown-up fruit salad that means business. SERVES 4

1 large, ripe mango (about 1lb 2oz/500g), diced

2 medium avocados (about 14oz/400g), diced

1¾ to 2¼oz (50 to 60g/about ½ bunch) watercress, leaves picked and stems finely chopped

1 to 2 red chiles, finely chopped (seeds and membranes removed if you want less heat)

1 small red onion (scant ¾ to ¾ cup/80 to 90g), diced

1 cup (25g/1 bunch) chives, finely chopped

Scant ½ cup (40g/a good handful) dried mango (not the soft, rehydrated kind), cut into thin strips

Sea salt, to taste

Juice of 3 limes (about 3 Tbsp)

Combine all the ingredients in a bowl and stir.

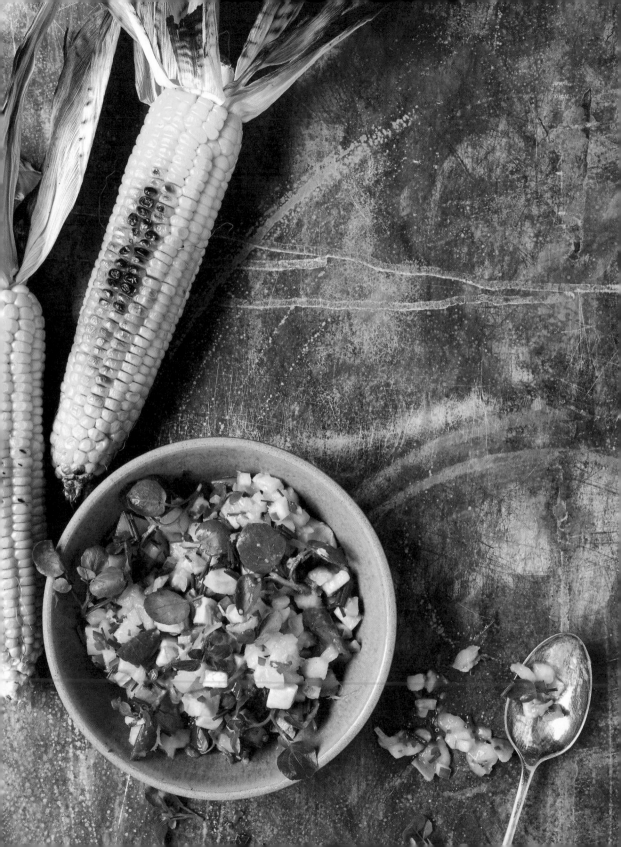

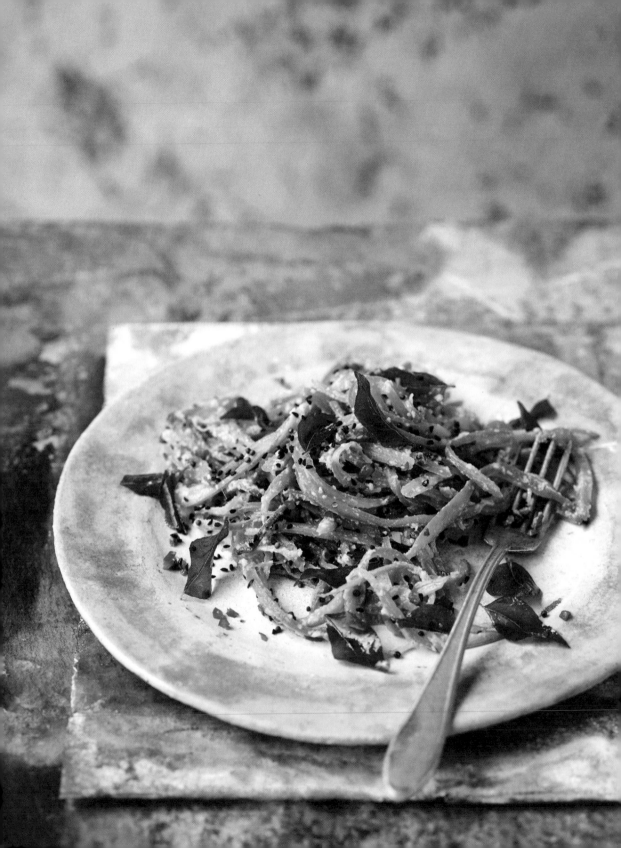

Curried string bean "tagliatelle"

Inspired by one of my favorite cuisines (Indian) and people (chef Rich LaMarita), this is a characterful side dish for when you need to add some pizzazz to a meal. Fresh curry leaves are now available at most major grocery stores and ethnic grocers. SERVES 4

15¾oz (450g) string beans, sliced lengthwise using a bean slicer, or in thirds lengthwise using a sharp knife, any strings removed

1 Tbsp coconut oil

½ tsp black mustard seeds

½ tsp cumin seeds

½ tsp black onion seeds (also called kalonji, nigella, black caraway, and black cumin seeds)

10 to 20 fresh curry leaves, depending on size

2 small or 1 large echalion (banana) shallots, halved lengthwise and sliced into half moons

1 Tbsp grated peeled ginger

1 garlic clove, mashed to a pulp with some coarse sea salt, using a mortar and pestle

1 red chile, finely chopped (seeds and membranes removed if you prefer it less spicy)

2 Tbsp creamed coconut (also called coconut manna or coconut butter)

Steam the beans (or boil in very little water) for 8 to 10 minutes, until tender and no longer crunchy. Refresh under cold running water.

While the beans are steaming, heat the coconut oil in a saucepan large enough to hold the beans, until hot but not smoking. Add the mustard seeds and cook until they just start to pop. Add the cumin and black onion seeds and fry until fragrant. Be careful not to let the spices burn, as they will taste bitter.

While the oil is still very hot, add the curry leaves. They should crackle almost immediately. Add the shallot and sauté for a few minutes before adding the ginger, garlic, and chile.

After a minute or so, add the cooked beans and creamed coconut and stir until the coconut has melted. Season to taste and serve.

Green celeriac mash

I never make plain potato mash any more. Since my aim is always to increase the amount of vegetables our family eats, I mix in mashed rutabaga, grated carrots, pureed cauliflower, and always something green. This version is a great way to up the greens intake without sacrificing flavor. SERVES 4

1 small celeriac (1¼ lb/550 to 600g), peeled and coarsely chopped

2 to 3 medium potatoes or white sweet potatoes (10½ to 12¼oz/300 to 350g), peeled and quartered

3 cups (120g) kale, thick stems removed, chopped

1 quantity of Roasted Garlic (page 154)

3 Tbsp butter

Sea salt

Cook the celeriac and potatoes separately in a little water until tender, adding more hot water after 10 minutes if necessary. Drain.

Meanwhile, steam the kale until wilted, then refresh under cold running water. Blitz in a food processor or finely chop using a very sharp knife.

Squeeze the roasted garlic from its skins into the potatoes, then pass the mixture through a potato ricer or food mill. Use a stick blender or food processor to blend the celeriac until smooth, then mix into the potato mash. Stir in the butter, chopped kale, and salt to taste.

Chargrilled zucchini and asparagus with tarragon dressing

I don't often grill or char vegetables; gentle cooking methods are considered most health supportive, as they preserve nutrients. But once in a while it is a lovely alternative to steaming, and the grill marks do add a note of festivity. If you cannot find fresh tarragon, use finely chopped, fresh marjoram or thyme, and add a pinch of ground anise. You can make the dressing and grill the vegetables in advance, but keep the elements separate until serving. SERVES 4

Steam the asparagus until just tender. Refresh under cold running water and blot dry with paper towels.

Heat a griddle pan until hot. Toss the zucchini slices and asparagus spears in a little grapeseed oil and place on the griddle in such a way as to achieve the most attractive grill pattern (allowing for one turn to create a crisscross effect).

Turn each zucchini slice once, and the asparagus spears a couple of times, making sure you don't turn or move the vegetables too early, or you may not get proper grill marks. A few minutes on each side should be about right. Set aside and keep warm. (Alternatively, you can cook the vegetables on a barbecue.)

Meanwhile, mash the garlic with a pinch of coarse sea salt, using a mortar and pestle. Scrape into a glass jar, add the oil, vinegar, and mustard with some pepper, screw the lid on tightly, and shake until the dressing is mixed well and emulsified. Stir in the herbs.

Toss the griddled vegetables in the dressing and arrange on a serving dish. Sprinkle over all the toasted almonds and serve immediately.

15¾oz (450g /1 bunch) asparagus (not the tender or fine version), tough part of stalks removed

2 medium zucchini (10½ to 12¼oz/ 300 to 350g), sliced diagonally into ⅜-in (1- to 1.5-cm) slices

Grapeseed oil, or cooking oil of your choice

Generous ⅓ cup (30g) slivered almonds, toasted in a dry frying pan until golden

FOR THE DRESSING
1 garlic clove

3 Tbsp extra-virgin olive oil

1 Tbsp tarragon vinegar, or cider vinegar

½ tsp Dijon mustard

1 Tbsp finely chopped tarragon leaves

1 Tbsp finely chopped chives

1 Tbsp finely chopped parsley

Coarse sea salt and freshly ground black pepper

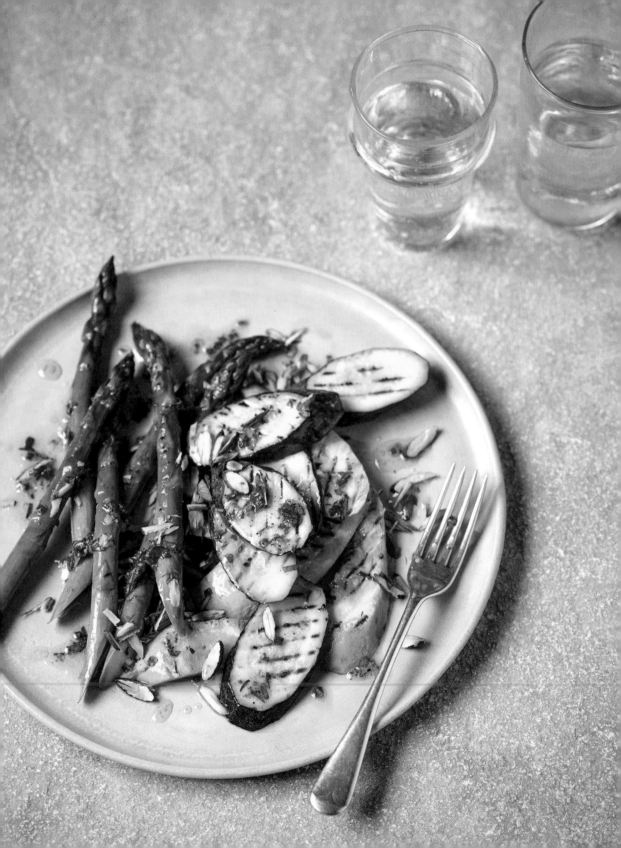

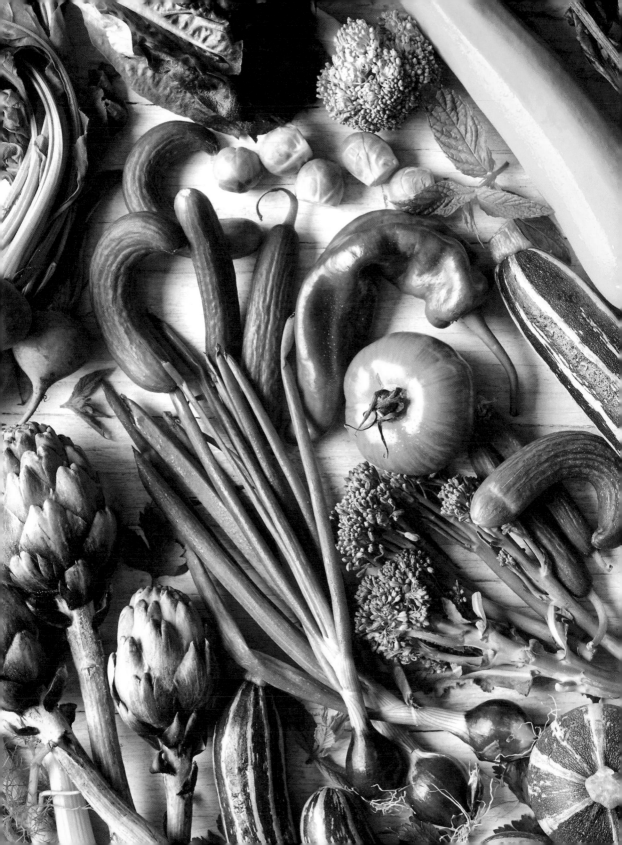

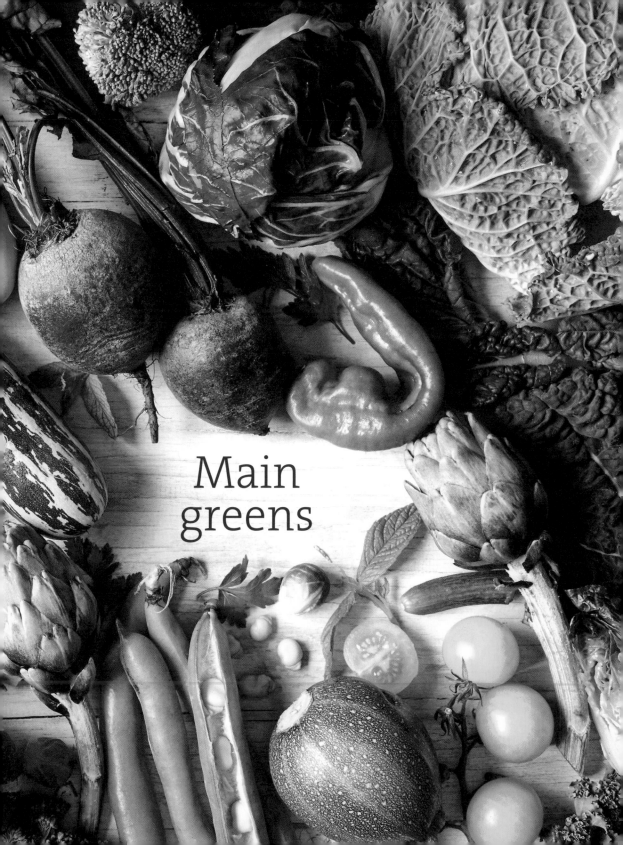

Main greens

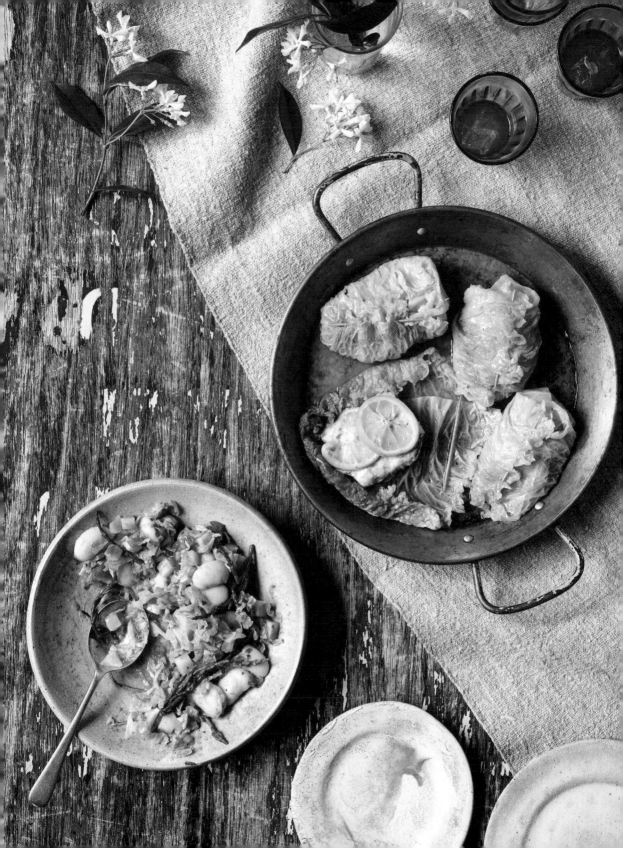

Savoy cabbage and snapper packages with braised lima beans

This is a lovely dish for when you are having friends around. Prep all your ingredients, then cook the veggies and fish at the same time. Choose small, but thick, pieces of fish (fleshy bourgeois red snapper and monkfish work well) and adjust the spiciness of your bean braise to suit your taste. Remember to remove 5 to 8 of the largest outer leaves of the cabbage before shredding, as you will need these to make your packages. SERVES 4

Heat the olive oil for the braised beans in a medium saucepan and sweat the onion with the salt over medium heat until soft and translucent. Add the celeriac, tomatoes, red pepper flakes, and a few Tbsp of the bean cooking liquid (or water), and braise, covered, for 10 to 15 minutes until the celeriac is tender.

Add the shredded cabbage and another Tbsp or two of the bean cooking liquid (or water) and cook for a few minutes until the cabbage is tender. Add the lima beans and samphire and cook for another 1 to 2 minutes. Stir in the parsley and keep warm.

Bring a large pan of salted water to a boil and blanch the large cabbage leaves for a minute or so until tender. Refresh in iced water or under cold running water, then pat dry.

Take the largest cabbage leaf and overlap the two halves to close the gap where the stalk would have been. Place a piece of fish, skin side down, on the leaf, season generously with salt and pepper, put a slice of butter on top, then 2 lemon slices next to each other, and wrap it up like a package, using toothpicks or kitchen string to secure the leaf. Repeat with the remaining cabbage leaves and fish ingredients, using 2 overlapping smaller leaves if one is not big enough to wrap the fish.

Place the packages in a saucepan that fits them snugly in a single layer. Pour in the wine, which should almost cover the packages, and bring to a boil. Reduce the heat and simmer for 10 to 15 minutes, or until the fish flakes easily when separated with a fork. You may want to turn the packages over halfway to ensure both sides are evenly cooked.

To serve, divide the bean mixture between four pasta bowls, drizzle with olive oil, remove the toothpicks from the fish packages, and place them on top. Alternatively, unwrap the fish and shred the cabbage leaf wrappers finely, then mix this into the beans before serving.

NOTE:
The braised beans alone also make a lovely vegan dish. Just add more cabbage and samphire to bulk it up.

FOR THE BRAISED BEANS

2 Tbsp olive oil, plus extra to serve

1 medium onion, diced

Pinch of sea salt

½ celeriac (12oz/300 to 350g), peeled and diced

4 plum or regular tomatoes (1⅔ to 1¾ cups/300 to 350g in total), blanched and skinned, quartered, seeded, and diced

Pinch of dried red pepper flakes, or to taste

½ savoy cabbage (5½ to 6⅓ cups/ 300 to 350g), finely shredded, setting aside outer leaves for the packages

2 cups (275g) cooked lima beans (about ½ cup/80g dried, see page 152), cooking liquid set aside

2½oz (60g/large handful) samphire, woody stalks removed (or asparagus, thinly sliced)

2 Tbsp finely chopped parsley

FOR THE FISH
5 to 8 large savoy cabbage leaves (see above), thick core removed and top part of leaf left intact

4 thick pieces of bourgeois snapper, 4¼ to 5oz (120 to 140g) each, pin-boned

4 thick slices of butter

8 slices of lemon

Generous 2 cups (500ml) dry white wine

Sea salt and freshly ground black pepper

Scallops with fennel relish and chunky parsnip mash

If you find fennel a little intimidating, this relish will shine a new light on it. Fennel has become one of my staple vegetables—grated into salads, roasted, lightly steamed. The recipe is a little time-consuming, as it requires lots of chopping, but it is worth the effort and, if you have any relish left over, it is also delicious with cheese and crackers or bean pâté crostini. If you can only find whole ancho chiles, grind them to a powder in a spice grinder or strong blender, or use a sharp knife to chop finely. SERVES 2 (OR 4 AS AN APPETIZER)

For the relish, peel the outer layer of the fennel bulb using a vegetable swivel peeler to get rid of any tough, stringy bits, then separate the layers and cut into small dice. Heat the olive oil in a pan and gently fry the fennel and onion with a pinch of salt until soft. Add the chili powder and fry for another 1 to 2 minutes.

Add the pear and all the citrus juices and simmer over medium heat, stirring regularly, until the juices have reduced to give a concentrated relish. Season with salt and pepper and stir in the fresh herbs. Set aside.

Meanwhile, cook the parsnips in a little water until tender, then drain and mash using a potato masher. Stir in the lamb's lettuce, olive oil, nutmeg, and some salt, then cover and keep warm.

Heat some butter in a cast-iron or other heavy-bottom frying pan over medium to high heat until frothy. Season the scallops with salt and black pepper before placing in the hot pan. Fry for 1 to 2 minutes, then turn them over, reduce the heat a little, and cook for another 1 to 3 minutes, depending on their size, or until just cooked. Take care not to overcook them.

Serve the scallops on a mound of parsnip mash, topped with the relish.

10½ to 12¼oz (300 to 350g/about 4) parsnips, trimmed and coarsely chopped

Handful of lamb's lettuce (mâche), coarsely chopped

Glug of extra-virgin olive oil

Good grating of nutmeg

Butter, for frying

8 scallops

FOR THE RELISH

1 fennel bulb (12¾ to 13½oz/360 to 380g), stalks discarded and fronds set aside for garnish

2 Tbsp extra-virgin olive oil

2 Tbsp finely chopped red onion

1 to 2 tsp ancho chili powder

1 large ripe, but not too soft, pear (about 7oz/200g), peeled and diced

3 Tbsp tangerine juice (1 tangerine)

3 Tbsp orange juice (about ½ large orange)

1 Tbsp lime juice (1 lime)

2 Tbsp very finely chopped mixture of dill, cilantro, and/or parsley

Sea salt and freshly ground black pepper

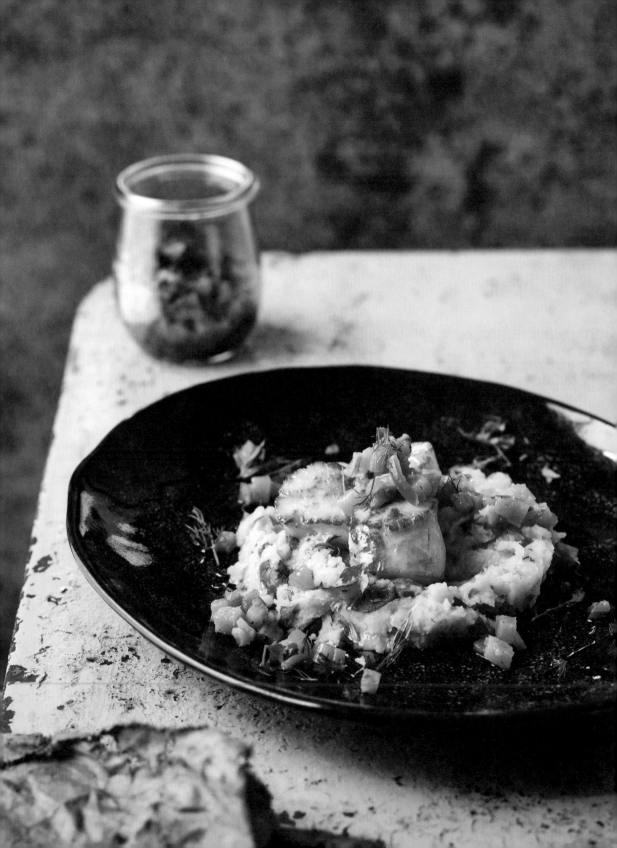

Lamb, mint, and cilantro burgers

This is one of my favorite ways with ground lamb. Serve with oven-baked, sweet potato fries, a large salad, and homemade tomato ketchup or a refreshing tzatziki. The bean sprouts add some crunch to the patties but if you are making these ahead to freeze, omit them. MAKES 4 EXTRA LARGE OR 8 MEDIUM PATTIES

Toast the cumin and coriander seeds in a dry, medium to hot frying pan for a couple of minutes until fragrant. Tip out, let cool slightly, then grind with a mortar and pestle or in a spice grinder. Set aside.

Chop the herbs as finely as possible. You could use a small food processor to do this, although I find it less efficient than doing it by hand. Set aside.

Grind the garlic and salt into a paste, using a mortar and pestle. Scrape this into a large mixing bowl and add all the other ingredients. Mix thoroughly with your hands and shape into 4 very large or 8 smaller patties.

Heat a little grapeseed or coconut oil in a large frying pan and fry the patties over medium to high heat until cooked to your liking— 5 to 7 minutes each side for the large patties, 4 to 5 minutes each side for the smaller ones.

1 tsp cumin seeds

1 tsp coriander seeds

¼ to ½oz (10 to 15g/small handful) mint, leaves only

1oz (25g/1 small bunch) parsley, leaves only

1oz (25g/1 small bunch) cilantro, largest stalks removed

1 garlic clove, coarsely chopped

Generous ½ tsp sea salt

½ cup (500g) ground lamb

Pinch of cayenne pepper

Generous grinding of black pepper

1 small onion, finely chopped

1 tsp Dijon mustard

1 scallion, very finely sliced

Large handful of mung bean sprouts, coarsely chopped (optional)

Grapeseed or coconut oil, for frying

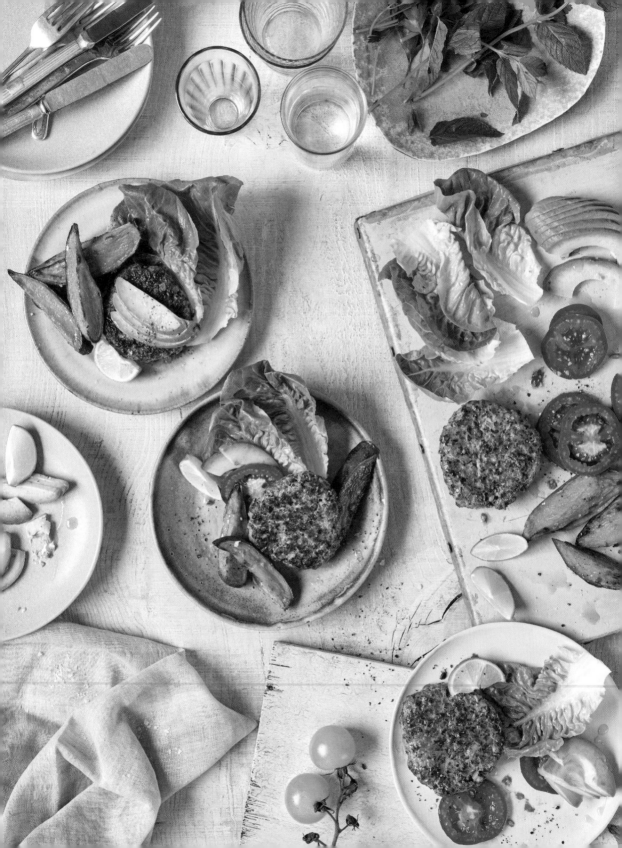

Portobello mushrooms with Tuscan kale and sweet potato

Tuscan kale is a cousin of curly kale and rather delicious; you can substitute one for the other in most recipes. Here I have opted for a mashed, soft mushroom filling, but you could just as well roast the sweet potato until crispy and the mushrooms until tender, roughly chop the cooked kale and mix everything together to pile on the baked mushrooms, then sprinkle the grated cheese over and broil for 5 to 10 minutes. SERVES 2 (OR 4 AS AN APPETIZER)

Preheat the oven to 350°F (180°C).

Remove the mushroom stalks using a small paring knife and season the caps with a little salt and pepper. Place them in an oven dish, gill-side up, that fits them snugly and set aside.

Heat the butter or oil in a saucepan and sweat the onion with a pinch of salt until soft and translucent. Stir in the garlic and, after another couple of minutes, add the chopped kale. Sauté until wilted and tender. You may want to add a splash of water to help this process along, but then be sure to cook until the saucepan is dry.

Transfer the kale and onion mixture to a food processor and process to finely chop (or do this using a large, sharp knife). Transfer to a bowl.

Mash the sweet potatoes with a little butter and salt, add to the kale mixture, then stir in the grated cheese, if using, and the corn.

Divide the mixture equally between the mushroom cavities and smooth the tops. Bake in the oven for 30 minutes or until the mushrooms are tender and the filling is crispy and golden on top.

Just before you are ready to serve, fry, poach or boil the eggs and season with salt and pepper.

Serve the stuffed mushrooms topped with an egg, and with a large green salad alongside.

4 large portobello mushrooms

A little butter or oil

1 medium onion, finely chopped

1 large garlic clove, finely chopped

3½oz (100g) Tuscan kale (or regular kale), thick stalks removed, leaves coarsely chopped

8¾oz (250g) peeled sweet potatoes, cut into medium dice and steamed until just tender

½ cup (50g) grated sharp cheddar cheese (optional)

1 ear of corn, kernels cut from the cob

4 eggs

Sea salt and freshly ground black pepper

Spinach and sardine dumplings

Oh my goodness! How much do I love these? They absolutely need to be eaten with lots of the tomato sauce, but as far as serving my family a moreish—and nutritious!—meal, this one is right up there with the best. The mixture or shaped dumplings can be prepared in advance and left in the refrigerator for a couple of days, making it a good fall-back option for busy evenings. Serve with a fresh green salad. MAKES ABOUT 20

Heat the oil, butter, or ghee in a pan, add the onion, and sauté until soft and translucent. Add the spinach and cook until wilted.

Squeeze the spinach to get rid of all the excess liquid. Either wear kitchen gloves to do this, or place the spinach in a colander and press against the sides with a large metal spoon (you can keep the water to feed your houseplants and herbs). This step is important; don't be tempted to skip it, or your dumplings will fall apart.

Put the dry spinach, sardines, and onion into a food processor and process to a smooth paste. Scrape this mixture into a bowl and mix in the nutmeg, garlic, quinoa or oat flakes, Parmesan, egg white, and a little salt (the Parmesan is salty) and pepper to taste.

If possible, cover the bowl and refrigerate for a few hours, to give the quinoa flakes time to soak up any excess liquid so the mixture is slightly easier to handle. (This is not essential if you are short of time.)

Use 2 Tbsp to form dumplings, scraping the mixture off the one with the other, or roll a small scoop of mixture between your hands to make a neat little ball.

Once you are ready to cook the dumplings, use a bamboo steamer, colander, or steamer insert in a saucepan with some shallow boiling water to steam them in batches, for about 10 minutes or until cooked through. You can brush some olive oil onto the insert to avoid the dumplings sticking to it.

Let the dumplings cool on a plate, covered, for a few minutes to firm them up, then serve with warmed Rich Tomato Sauce, a drizzle of good olive oil, and grated Parmesan.

A little olive oil, butter, ghee or coconut oil

1 medium onion, diced

14oz (400g) spinach, washed and roughly torn

4¼-oz (120-g) can of sardines in olive oil, drained

1 tsp freshly grated nutmeg

2 garlic cloves, finely chopped

1 cup (100g) quinoa flakes (or fine oat flakes)

Scant 1 cup (60g) grated Parmesan cheese

1 egg white, lightly whisked

Sea salt and freshly ground black pepper

TO SERVE
1 quantity of Rich Tomato Sauce (page 153), warmed

Good olive oil

Grated Parmesan cheese

Millet and watercress sushi
with creamy aduki bean paste

Few things give me more pleasure than homemade sushi. It is such a satisfactory process and allows for complete customization, each roll providing a fresh canvas for the artist in the kitchen. If your first try looks a little messy, take heart —you will need only a few attempts to perfect your technique and, with all these deliciously nutritious ingredients, you won't mind practicing. SERVES 4 TO 6

For the paste, blend all the ingredients together in a blender or food processor until smooth, then set aside.

Toast the millet in a dry pan until it smells like popcorn. Add the water and salt and bring to a boil. Reduce the heat, cover, and simmer, stirring occasionally, until soft and sticky, 25 to 30 minutes.

Meanwhile, whisk together the brown rice vinegar and honey. Pour the mixture over the cooked millet, spread it out on an oven tray, and let cool just slightly; you want it still warm to assemble the rolls.

Place a nori sheet on a sushi mat, shiny side down and the ridges running parallel to the bamboo. Wet your fingertips and spread about 6 heaping Tbsp millet on the nori sheet, leaving ¾ in (2 cm) free at the top and the bottom of the sheet. Use your fingertips to press the millet down on the nori very firmly. Millet does not have the same stickiness as rice, so you need to use some elbow grease here.

Spread 1 Tbsp bean paste over the lower half of the millet, then place a few pepper sticks, some asparagus spears, 2 avocado strips, and a few watercress sprigs on top.

Lift the bottom edge of your sushi mat and roll away from you, guiding the nori sheet downward and tucking it in around the filling to form a roll. Continue rolling the mat away from you until the nori is used up around the roll.

Turn the mat around and pull gently on the loose end while pressing the roll away from you to secure its shape. Use a very sharp knife to cut into 5 or 6 slices. Serve with the ginger, wasabi, and shoyu dipping sauce.

NOTE:
Always try to buy naturally fermented soy sauce (shoyu), which is traditionally made by fermenting soybeans, water, wheat, and a special starter fungus. Because this can take up to a few years, many producers now cook the soybeans with hydrochloric acid, thereby eliminating the fermentation step, which is necessary in making soy digestible and beneficial.

6 nori sheets

1 red bell pepper (about 3½oz/100g), cored and cut into 2-in (5-cm) sticks

1 small bunch (3½oz/100g) of slender asparagus stalks, trimmed and lightly steamed

1 avocado, peeled and cut into thin strips

1 small bunch of watercress, thick stems removed and leaves snipped

FOR THE PASTE
1 cup (150g) cooked aduki beans (¼ cup/50g uncooked, see page 152)

1½ Tbsp grated peeled ginger

1 Tbsp tahini

2 Tbsp lemon juice (about 1 lemon)

1 Tbsp maple syrup

Pinch of cayenne pepper

1 small garlic clove

Sea salt, to taste

FOR THE MILLET
Scant 1⅔ cups (300g) millet, rinsed

3 cups (750ml) water

Large pinch of sea salt

¼ cup (60ml) brown rice vinegar

1 Tbsp runny honey

TO SERVE
Naturally pickled ginger

Wasabi paste

Shoyu (or tamari) and rice vinegar dipping sauce (mixed together in a 2:1 ratio)

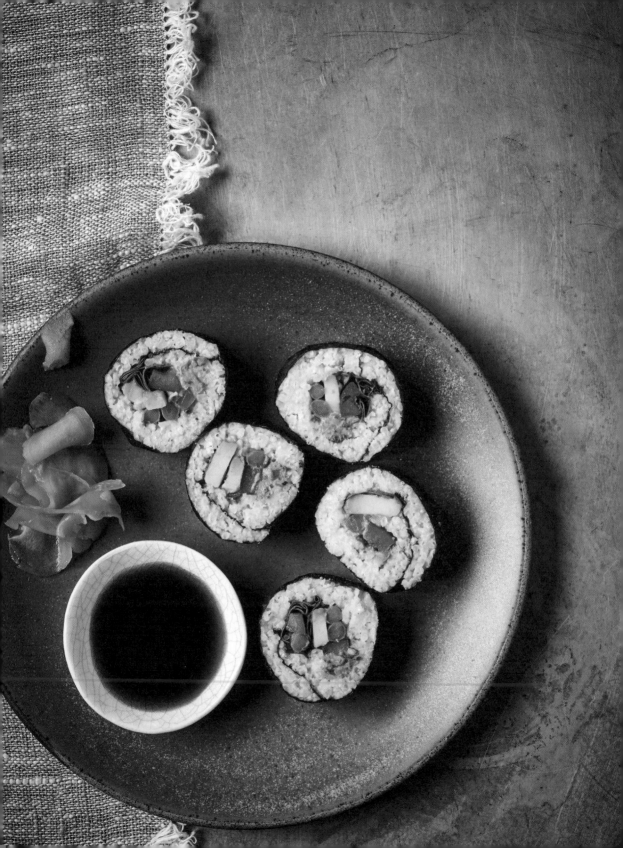

Barley and mustard greens risotto

Most people, myself included, love a good risotto—a creamy, unctuous dish that comfort-food dreams are made of. But what risotto boasts in yum factor, it lacks on the nutrition front. Here is a toothier version that will hopefully also satisfy those looking for a little more green in their lives. Remember to soak your barley for at least 8 hours before you plan to make this. Mustard greens and arugula are pungent and spicy leaves, so opt for spinach instead if you prefer a milder taste. Serve with extra grated or shaved Parmesan and a tomato salad. SERVES 2 (OR 4 AS A SIDE DISH OR APPETIZER)

Sauté the onion in some butter, ghee, olive oil, or coconut oil with a pinch of sea salt over medium heat until soft and translucent. Add the leeks and continue to cook until tender.

Turn up the heat and add the barley. Add a ladleful of broth at a time, stirring until it is completely absorbed before adding the next ladleful. Continue doing this until the barley is tender, for about 25 to 35 minutes, adding salt and pepper to taste along the way and stirring regularly. Remember that barley will never be soft and squidgy; even when cooked, the kernels remain chewy.

Spoon 2 to 3 Tbsp of the tender barley and the pulp of the Roasted Garlic into a blender (or tall container if using a stick blender), and add just enough hot broth (about ¼ cup/60ml) to be able to blend into a creamy paste. If it is too sticky or stodgy, add some more broth.

Now scrape the paste, which will help make the risotto creamy, back into the risotto pan, and stir in the mustard leaves, parsley, petits pois, and Parmesan. Cover with a lid for a few minutes or until the leaves have wilted and the peas are cooked. Adjust the seasoning.

Turn off the heat and stir in the egg yolk. The residual heat from the barley will cook the yolk and make for a creamier end result. Sprinkle over some pea shoots and serve immediately.

1 medium onion, diced

Butter, ghee, or olive, or coconut oil, for frying

2 medium leeks, halved lengthwise and sliced into half-moons

Generous 1 cup (220g) pearl barley, soaked overnight, or for 8 to 12 hours, then rinsed

2 to 3 cups (500 to 750ml) fresh chicken or vegetable broth, kept just below simmering

1 quantity of Roasted Garlic (page 154)

1 bunch (about 1¾oz/50g) of mustard leaves, arugula, or baby leaf spinach, coarsely chopped

¾ cup (20g/small bunch) parsley, leaves only, finely chopped

¾ cup (110g) fresh or frozen petits pois

¾ cup (50g) grated Parmesan cheese, plus extra for serving

1 egg yolk, lightly whisked

Sea salt and freshly ground black pepper

Pea shoots, to serve (optional)

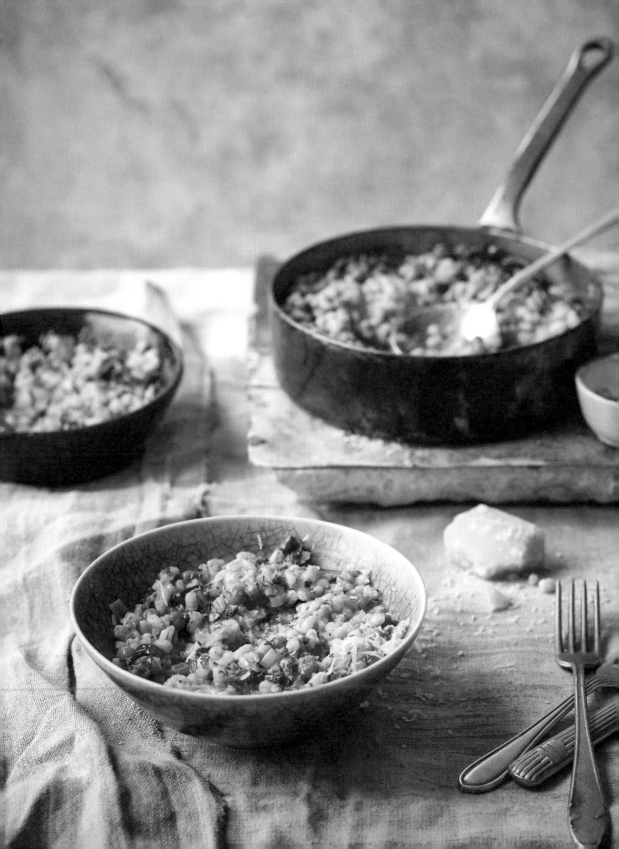

Grain-free cauliflower "pizza" with chard and olives

Thanks to popular diets such as the Paleo diet and other grain-free diets, we have come to love cauliflower for its versatility. Not only can it impersonate couscous, be turned into risotto and used instead of macaroni in mac 'n' cheese, it can also become a nutritious grain-free flour, by squeezing every last drop of liquid from it. SERVES 2

Preheat a pizza stone (or heavy, flat baking tray) in the oven at 430°F (220°C). Blitz the cauliflower in a food processor until it resembles couscous, then steam in a strainer or steamer over a small amount of simmering water until tender. Let cool completely.

Spoon the cauliflower into a nut milk bag or several layers of cheesecloth and squeeze out all the liquid. You should end up with 7oz (200g) cauliflower "flour." This process can seem laborious, but is essential.

In a bowl, combine the "flour" and the remaining ingredients for the base, with a pinch of salt and pepper, and mix well.

Using your hands, press the dough onto a large piece of oiled baking parchment, to about ¼in (5mm) thick. Slide the baking parchment onto the hot pizza stone or baking tray in the oven and bake for 10 minutes. Remove from the oven, flip over, and peel off the parchment. Return to the oven by sliding onto the pizza stone or baking sheet directly, then bake for another 5 minutes or until golden and crispy around the edges.

While the base is baking, gently cook the onion in a pan with some oil or ghee and a pinch of salt over low heat. Once soft and translucent, turn up the heat to medium and add the tomatoes. When the tomatoes start to soften, add the garlic and cook for another 2 to 3 minutes. Add the chard and cook until wilted. Stir in the olives, remove from the heat, and keep warm.

When the base is cooked, remove from the oven and let stand for a couple of minutes before topping with the chard mixture. Sprinkle on some crumbly cheese and chili oil, if using.

NOTE:
The steamed cauliflower does take a long time to cool down, so if it's more convenient, prepare the "flour" in advance and keep refrigerated until ready to continue with the recipe.

FOR THE BASE

1 medium cauliflower, florets only

1 medium egg, lightly beaten

1 tsp dried mixed Italian herbs (oregano, marjoram, basil, etc.)

Scant ¼ cup (20g) ground almonds

¼ cup (20g) finely grated Parmesan cheese (optional)

Sea salt and freshly ground black pepper

FOR THE TOPPING

1 large red onion, cut in half through the core, peeled, and sliced

Coconut oil, ghee, or high-quality extra-virgin olive oil

14oz (400g) cherry tomatoes, halved

2 garlic cloves, pressed or mashed

7oz (200g) chard, chopped into small bite-size pieces (chop stalks separately if thick)

Large handful (about ½ cup/50g) of pitted kalamata olives

TO SERVE (OPTIONAL)
Crumbly goat cheese

Chili olive oil

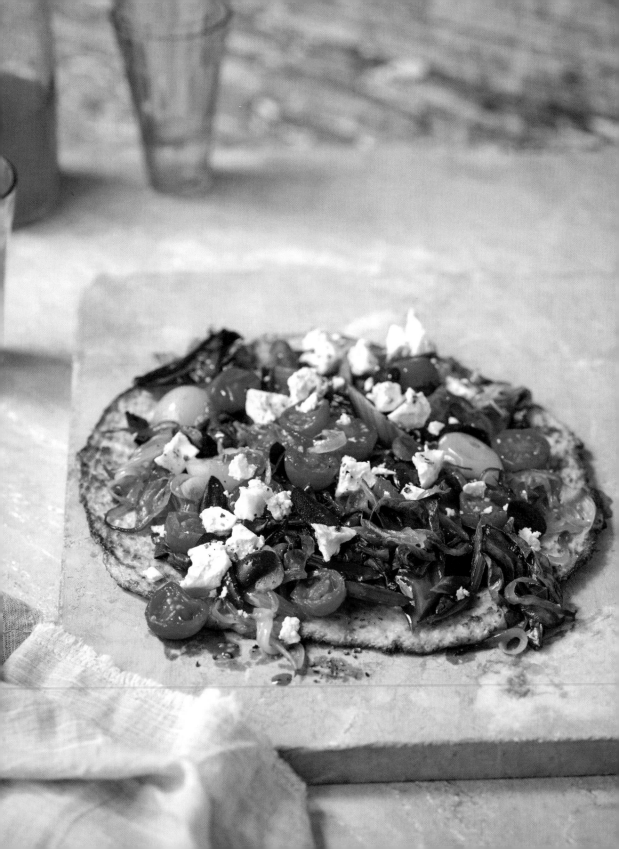

Collard greens lasagna

As with most lasagna recipes, this one does take a little time, but it will feed a large crowd (or your family twice!) and it's a pleasure to know you have something ready to pop in the oven as soon as you get home from that long walk or exhausting shopping trip. The béchamel is made with butternut squash, so it comes out a lovely bright color. SERVES 6

For the butternut béchamel, cook the butternut squash in a little water until tender. Drain and mash. You should end up with about 1½ cups (350g) mashed butternut squash.

Mix the arrowroot or kuzu with enough of the cold milk to dissolve it and form a thin paste. In a blender or with a stick blender, blend the rest of the milk with the mashed butternut mash until smooth.

Transfer the mixture to a small saucepan with the bay leaf and arrowroot or kuzu paste and heat, stirring continuously, until the mixture is simmering and starts to thicken. Cook for 1 to 2 minutes, then remove from the heat, generously season with salt and pepper, and set aside. If the sauce is still too thin, add a little more kuzu or arrowroot dissolved in milk.

For the spring greens, heat some butter, or coconut or olive oil in a medium saucepan and sweat the onion with a pinch of salt. Add the collard greens and sauté until wilted. Remove from the heat and let cool. Meanwhile, preheat the oven to 350°F (180°C).

Put the ricotta, thyme leaves, eggs, and sausage meat (or mushrooms) into a food processor and add the cold greens. Process until smooth.

To assemble, boil enough water to cover the bottom of a dish or shallow bowl that will fit 1 lasagna sheet. Steep the first lasagna sheet in the hot water for at least 10 seconds, or until it starts to soften. Remove and place in a medium ovenproof dish. Repeat until your first layer of sheets is complete. Break a sheet in half to fill any edges or corners if necessary.

Spread half the collard greens mixture over the lasagna, then half the Basic Tomato Sauce and half the butternut sauce. Repeat the process for the lasagna sheets with the second layer and repeat the layering of the sauces.

Top with the grated cheese, if using, and bake for 1 hour. Let stand for 10 minutes before serving, to give the lasagna a chance to firm up.

6 to 8 dried wholewheat or spinach lasagna sheets

1 quantity of Basic Tomato Sauce (page 153)

Scant 1 cup (100g) grated Gruyère cheese (optional)

FOR THE BUTTERNUT BÉCHAMEL
½ medium butternut squash, peeled, halved, seeded, and coarsely chopped

2½ Tbsp arrowroot powder or crushed kuzu root starch, or 2 tsp cornstarch

1½ cups (375ml) milk of your choice (I use fresh almond milk)

1 bay leaf

Sea salt and freshly ground black pepper

FOR THE COLLARD GREENS
Butter, or coconut or olive oil

1 medium onion, diced

2 heads of collard greens (about 1lb 4oz/600g), thick stalks removed, leaves coarsely chopped

Generous 1 cup (250g) ricotta

1½ Tbsp thyme leaves

2 eggs, lightly beaten

14oz (400g) sausage meat (from about 6 sausages) or 14oz (400g) cooked mushrooms

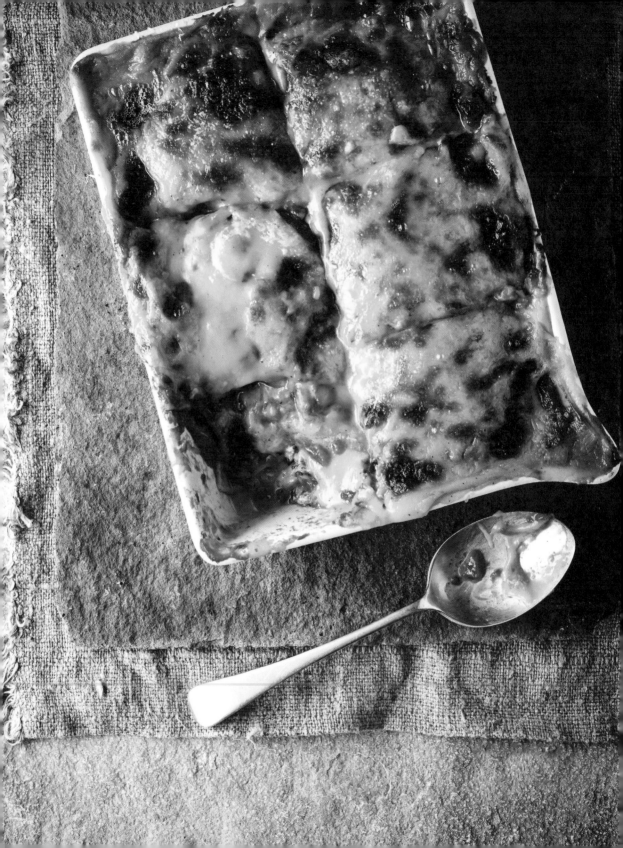

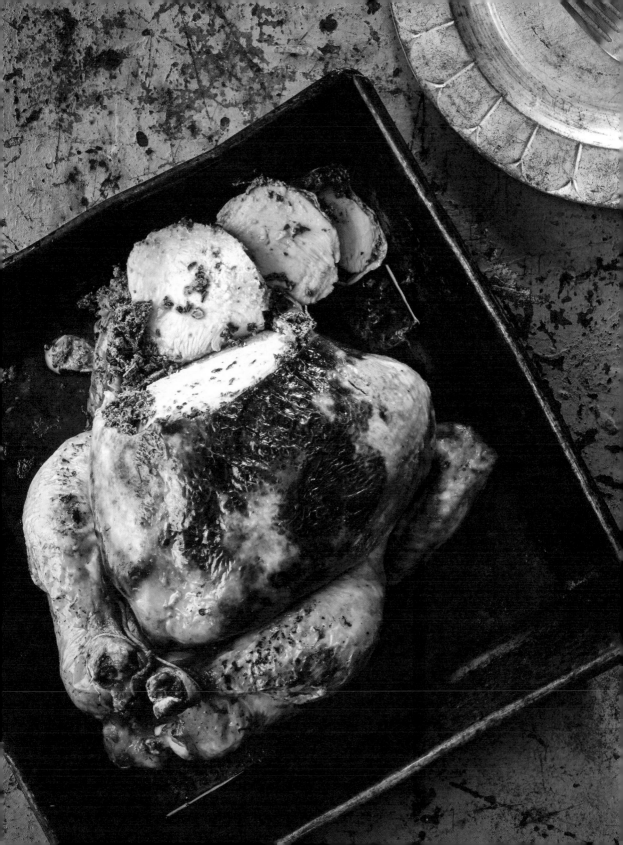

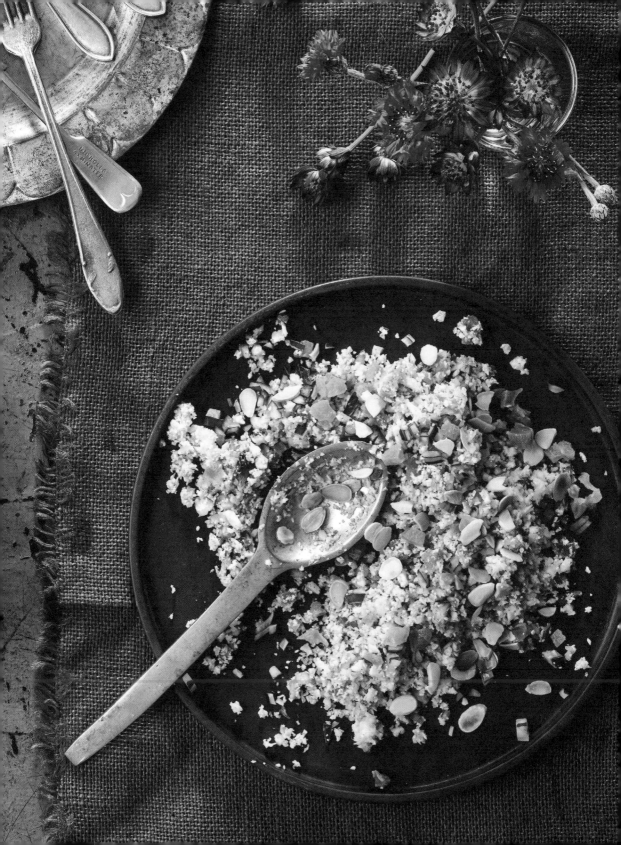

Kale and lemon-stuffed chicken with cauliflower "couscous"

Nothing quite beats a roast chicken. This is an interesting version and even hard-nosed antiveg campaigners have asked for second helpings. Although a staple in the "living foods" circles for the longest of times, raw cauliflower "couscous" has never been a favorite of mine. My tummy is a little sensitive and too many raw foods, especially of the cruciferous kind, tend to wreak havoc. However, I did not want to give up, which is how the recipe for this couscous came about. SERVES 6 TO 8

Preheat the oven to 350°F (180°C).

Wash the kale, discarding any tough stalks, and put in a big saucepan with a little water. Cook over medium heat until wilted, then transfer to a colander and let drain and cool before squeezing out any excess water.

Toast the cumin and coriander seeds in dry frying pan until fragrant. Grind in a spice grinder or with a mortar and pestle.

Put the kale, ground seeds, preserved lemon peel, and salt into a food processor and process until finely ground. Stir through the goat curd.

Put the chicken into a roasting pan. Gently slide your fingers between the skin and the flesh of the chicken to create pockets and fill these pockets with the kale mixture. I usually loosen the skin on the breasts and around the legs, pressing filling into all the nooks and crannies. That way you should be able to use it all up.

Put the cinnamon, garlic, lemon, and onion quarters into the cavity of the chicken, cover the roasting pan with foil and roast for 35 minutes. Remove the foil and roast for another 35 to 45 minutes, or until the juices run clear when the thickest part of a thigh is pricked with a skewer. Let rest, covered, for at least 10 minutes.

While the chicken is roasting, blitz the cauliflower in a food processor until it resembles couscous. Stir-fry the cauliflower couscous in a medium to hot pan with a little butter or oil until tender, 5 to 8 minutes.

Mix the cooked cauliflower in a serving bowl with the remaining couscous ingredients, except the slivered almonds, then sprinkle slivered almonds on top and serve with the chicken.

PHOTOGRAPH ON PAGES 96 TO 97

7oz (200g) kale

1 tsp cumin seeds

1 tsp coriander seeds

1 medium preserved lemon (1½ to 1¾oz/40 to 50g), flesh removed and peel finely chopped

1 scant tsp sea salt

⅔ cup (150g) goat curd or rindless soft goat cheese

1 large chicken (about 4½lb/2kg), giblets removed

1 cinnamon stick

2 garlic cloves, peeled and crushed

1 lemon, washed and pricked with a skewer in several places, then quartered lengthwise

1 medium onion, peeled and quartered

FOR THE CAULIFLOWER "COUSCOUS"
1 large cauliflower (1¼ to 1½lb/600 to 700g), separated into florets

1 small red onion, finely chopped and soaked in cold water for 15 minutes

½ cup (70g/about 10) preservative-free dried apricots, diced

1 tsp ras-el-hanout (see page 155)

¾-in (2-cm) piece of fresh turmeric root, grated (or ½ tsp ground)

1½ Tbsp butter (optional)

2 Tbsp extra-virgin olive oil

Juice of 1 lemon

Pinch of sea salt

⅔ cup (50g) slivered almonds, toasted

Broccoli and brown rice bake
with soft-boiled eggs

*The success of this dish rests on using the most flavorsome broth.
If you are not vegetarian, I would recommend chicken broth,
otherwise be sure to use a veggie broth with a deep flavor. If you
have any leftovers, add to 1 to 2 whisked eggs and stir in 1 to 2 Tbsp
flour to make little fritters.* SERVES 4 (OR 6 AS A SIDE DISH)

Preheat the oven to 350°F (180°C).

Put all the ingredients, except the broccoli and chives, into a
medium ovenproof dish or Dutch oven that has a lid, and stir to
combine. Cover and bake in the oven for 45 to 50 minutes.

Meanwhile, cut the large and smaller stalks of the broccoli into
small dice and separate the florets into small bits.

Carefully remove the dish from the oven, add the broccoli stems,
and give the contents a good stir. Cover and return to the oven.
After 10 minutes, add the florets, give it another stir, ensuring
the top layer of rice is mixed under, and bake for another
5 to 10 minutes.

Remove from the oven and test the rice; it should be tender and
sticky, almost like risotto. If it is still a little *al dente*, return to the
oven for another 5 minutes.

Remove from the oven and let stand, covered, for 10 minutes
before sprinkling with the chives and serving with soft-boiled
eggs and a grating of Parmesan, if you like.

Scant 3 cups (680ml) hot vegetable or
chicken broth

1 large onion, chopped into small dice

2 garlic cloves, finely chopped

1 Tbsp extra-virgin olive oil

1 heaping tsp sea salt

1 heaping tesp mixed dried *herbes
de Provence*

1 tsp ground turmeric

1 tsp ground paprika

1 tsp ground coriander

½ cup (60g/about 10 halves) sundried
tomatoes in olive oil, cut into thin strips

1⅔ cups (300g) short-grain brown
rice, rinsed

1 small head (10½ to 11¼oz/300 to 320g)
of broccoli

Handful of chives, finely chopped

TO SERVE
Soft-boiled eggs

Freshly grated Parmesan cheese
(optional)

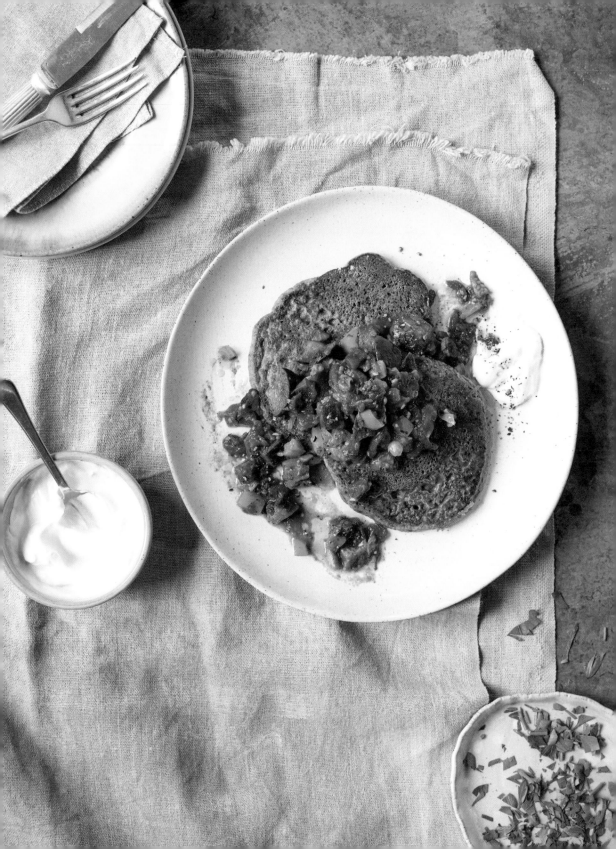

Chickpea and chard pancakes with eggplant stew

Another favorite in our household, chickpea pancakes work well with many toppings and flavors. Timing is important, as the batter needs to stand for at least a few hours before cooking the pancakes, and the pan needs to be preheated. They are also best served while they are still hot and crispy, so we usually eat them in shifts. SERVES 4

To make the pancake batter, put the gram flour in a bowl, make a well in the center, and whisk in the coconut oil, a large pinch of salt, and most of the water until you have a thick batter. Add more water if necessary, then set aside for 4 hours.

Preheat the oven to 430°F (220°C).

Heat the olive oil in a saucepan and sauté the onion for the batter with a pinch of salt over medium heat until soft and translucent. Add the rosemary and fry for another minute before scraping into a food processor and setting aside.

Tip the chard stalks into the pan, add a tiny bit of water, cover, and "steam" until tender. Add the chard leaves and cook, uncovered, until wilted, for about 1 minute or longer if the leaves are very coarse, and the saucepan is dry.

Add this mixture to the food processor (no need to squeeze it out first), process until very fine and set aside. Stir into the chickpea batter just before you cook the pancakes.

For the eggplant stew, heat some fat of your choice in a saucepan and sauté the red onion with a pinch of salt for a few minutes. Add the garlic and eggplant and increase the heat a little. As soon as the eggplant is halfway to being tender, add the chopped tomatoes, thyme leaves, chopped bell pepper, and cayenne pepper, cover, and cook, stirring occasionally for 20 to 30 minutes until the eggplant is soft but not squishy.

Add the orange juice and parsley, simmer for another minute, season, remove from the heat, and keep warm.

Meanwhile, place one large or two smaller cast-iron skillets or heavy-bottom stainless steel pans in the oven with a large piece of ghee or coconut oil. As soon as it is very hot (but not smoking) and the fat covers the bottom in a noticeable layer, remove from the oven and ladle enough of the chickpea mixture into the pan(s) to make several small, or one large pancake. You will hear a sizzling sound. Slide back into the oven and bake for 10 to 20 minutes or until very crispy around the edges and slightly golden on top. Repeat with the remaining pancake mixture until it is all used up. Serve straight from the oven with the eggplant stew and Greek yogurt or Vegan Greek-style "Yogurt."

FOR THE PANCAKES

2⅔ cups (240g) gram flour (chickpea flour)

1½ Tbsp liquid coconut oil

1¼ cups (310ml) tepid water

A little olive oil

1 medium onion, chopped

1 heaping Tbsp finely chopped rosemary

7oz (200g) chard, thick stalks cut out and finely chopped, leaves torn into smaller pieces

Ghee or coconut oil, for frying

Sea salt

FOR THE EGGPLANT STEW

Coconut oil, butter, or extra-virgin olive oil

1 large red onion, finely chopped

2 garlic cloves, finely chopped

About 1lb to 1lb 2oz (480 to 500g/about 2 medium) eggplants, cut into ⅝-in (1.5cm) dice

About 1lb to 1lb 2oz (480 to 500g/ about 5) large tomatoes, blanched, skinned, fibrous core removed, chopped

1 heaping Tbsp thyme leaves, finely chopped

1 orange bell pepper, cut into small dice

Pinch of cayenne pepper

3 Tbsp freshly squeezed orange juice (about 1 medium orange)

1 cup (25g/1 small bunch) flat-leaf parsley, finely chopped

Greek yogurt or Vegan Greek-style "Yogurt" (page 157), to serve

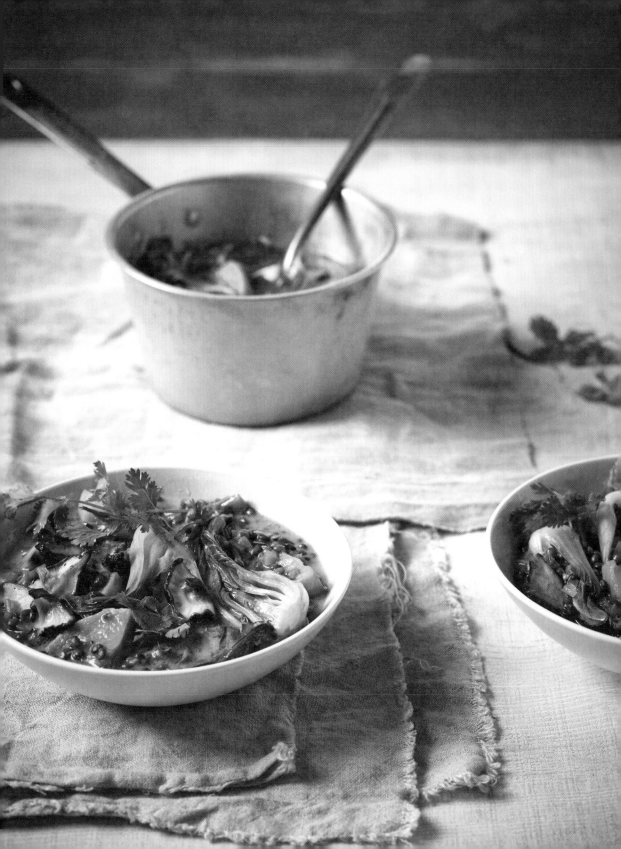

Lentil, bok choy, and mushroom curry

This is one of my favorite midweek suppers. I often increase the quantity of bok choy, as I love the taste and the shocks of green. It can be made ahead and kept in the refrigerator for a few days, but I would reserve the bok choy leaves, cilantro, and ginger juice to be added to the heated curry just before serving. SERVES 3 TO 4

Preheat the oven to 350°F (180°C).

Toss the butternut dice in some salt, pepper, and oil, then roast in the oven for 40 to 50 minutes until tender and golden, turning the pieces over using a spatula after about 20 minutes.

Meanwhile, heat a little oil in a large pan, add the onion, and sauté until soft and translucent. Add the garlic and cook for another couple of minutes, then tip into a small bowl. Heat a little more oil, add the mushrooms, and fry, in batches, over medium to high heat until nicely browned and tender.

Add the lentils, red pepper flakes, coconut milk, and broth, and simmer, uncovered, for about 15 minutes until the lentils are almost tender. Add the bok choy stems, increase the heat to high, and cook for another 5 minutes, or until the sauce has thickened and is sticky around the edges of the pan.

Add the bok choy leaves and, as soon as they have wilted, add the ginger juice to taste, and the cilantro. Top with the roasted squash and serve immediately, either as it is, or with cauliflower "couscous" or brown basmati rice cooked with sliced ginger, ground turmeric, and cloves.

1 large butternut squash, peeled, halved, seeded, and flesh chopped into large dice

Grapeseed, coconut, macadamia, or other oil

1 large onion, finely diced

3 medium garlic cloves, finely chopped

1 punnet (4¼ to 4½oz/120 to 130g) oyster mushrooms, cleaned and cut into bite-size pieces

1 punnet (4¼ to 4½oz/120 to 130g) shiitake mushrooms, cleaned, stalks removed, and thickly sliced

½ cup (100g) Puy lentils, soaked overnight, then rinsed

Large pinch of dried red pepper flakes, or to taste

14-oz (400ml) can coconut milk

½ cup (125ml) vegetable broth

7oz (200g) bok choy, stems thickly sliced and leaves coarsely chopped

Juice from 2-in (5-cm) piece of ginger, grated and juice squeezed out (use a nut milk bag, cheesecloth, or your hands)

Large handful (1½ to 2 cups/40 to 50g) of cilantro, finely chopped

Sea salt and freshly ground black pepper

Cape Malay-style mutton curry

South African cuisine is a wonderful mishmash of cultural influences and the ready access to tasty fresh produce in most parts of the country is a cook's dream. A personal highlight is the Cape Malay heritage with its richly flavored and Indonesian-inspired dishes. If you are vegetarian, replace the meat with chickpeas and roasted pumpkin or butternut squash. This recipe does make quite a lot, but it seems a waste to make a smaller portion if you are going to go to all the effort. Any leftovers can be frozen. SERVES 6 TO 8

Grind the fennel and coriander seeds, red pepper flakes, peppercorns, cardamom, and cumin seeds in a mortar and pestle (or use a spice grinder) until finely ground.

Heat some oil in a shallow pan, large enough to fit all the pieces of meat, and brown the meat on all sides. Remove from the pan and set aside.

In the same pan, sweat the onion until soft and translucent. Add the ginger and cook for another few minutes. Add the ground spices, turmeric, garam masala, cinnamon stick, cloves, and bay leaves, and stir for a couple of minutes. Stir in the remaining ingredients except the spinach and pineapple, and tuck the pieces of meat into the sauce.

Cover and simmer for at least 2 hours, or until the meat is very tender, gently turning over the pieces of meat once or twice during cooking.

When the meat is close to falling off the bone, skim off excess fat, carefully transfer the meat to a serving dish, and check the sauce for any small bones that may have fallen off during cooking. Stir the spinach and pineapple into the sauce and simmer, covered, for another 10 minutes, or until the spinach is wilted and the pineapple is cooked.

Serve the meat on turmeric rice with the sauce, topped with banana slices and dry unsweetened coconut.

NOTE:
The curry's flavors develop over time, so leave it in the refrigerator for a day or two before serving, if you can, and enjoy the thought of having another meal ready for later that same week.

3 tsp fennel seeds

1½ tsp coriander seeds

1 to 2 tsp dried red pepper flakes, to taste

½ tsp black peppercorns

Seeds of 10 cardamom pods

2 tsp cumin seeds

Grapeseed or coconut oil, for frying

2½lb (1.2kg) mutton (or lamb) neck pieces, bone in

1 large onion, finely chopped

1 Tbsp grated peeled ginger

2 tsp ground turmeric (or 3 tsp freshly grated root)

1 Tbsp garam masala

1 cinnamon stick

4 cloves

2 bay leaves

2 tsp sea salt

2 x 14-oz (400-g) cans of chopped tomatoes

2 Tbsp tomato paste

2 to 3 garlic cloves, finely chopped

2 tsp brown sugar

2 Tbsp cider vinegar

7 to 8¾oz (200 to 250g) baby spinach

1 small pineapple, flesh cut into cubes

TO SERVE
Turmeric rice

2 ripe but firm medium bananas, sliced

Dry unsweetened coconut

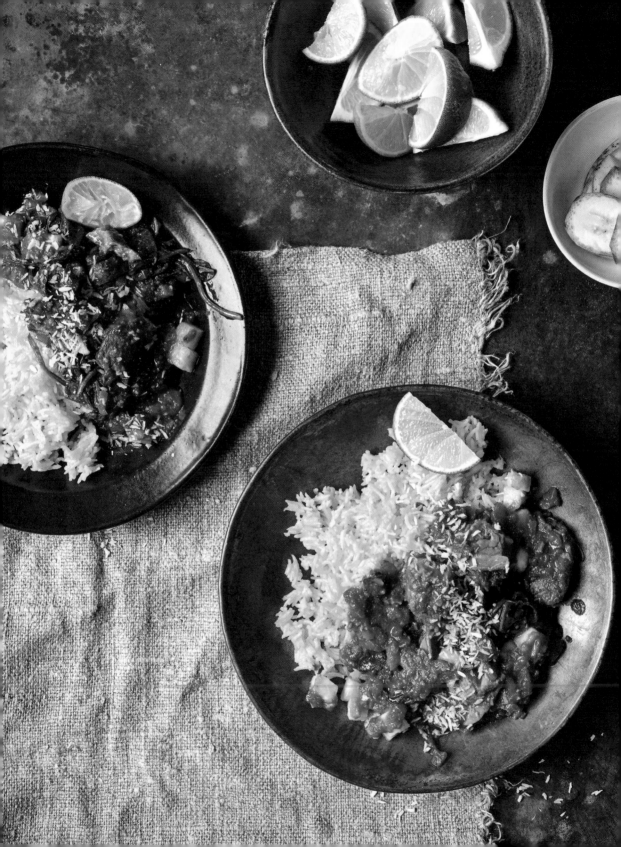

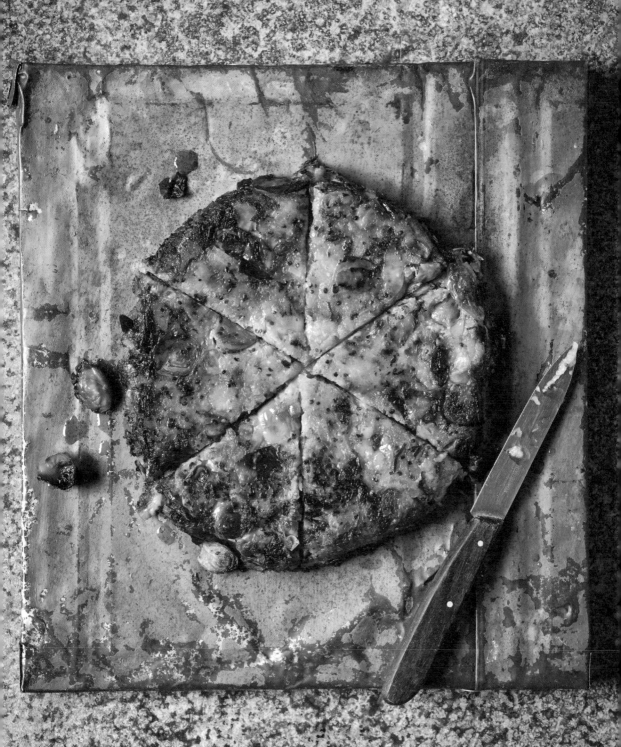

Brussels sprout, leek, and potato cake

This is a delicious way to prepare a bunch of humble vegetables. Serve with sour cream or Greek yogurt, sustainably sourced caviar (try Mottra caviar) and smoked wild salmon, for a festive occasion, or with roasted tomatoes and a large mixed salad for lunch or a light supper. It is also terrific as a brunch dish with wilted spinach and poached eggs. SERVES 4 TO 6

Preheat the oven to 350°F (180°C).

Use a small knife to cut a cross into each potato (or prick a few times with a fork) and roast for 1 to 1½ hours, or until just tender. As soon as they are cool enough to handle, scoop out the insides and mash with a fork, leaving them very lumpy. Increase the oven temperature to 430°F (220°C).

While the potatoes are baking, heat a third of the butter in a medium (about 9½-in/24-cm) ovenproof frying pan and fry the sage for a minute or two. Add the leek and a large pinch of salt, and cook over medium heat until tender. Scrape into a large bowl and set aside.

Increase the heat in the pan, add half the remaining butter, shake off any excess water from the sprouts, and sauté until nicely browned. Scrape into the bowl with the leeks. Add the crushed potatoes to the bowl with some salt, pepper, and the mustard, and mix well.

Heat the remaining butter in the pan and, once it is very hot, spoon in the potato mixture (you should hear it sizzle) and press it down with the back of a large spoon until it is smooth and compact. Transfer to the oven and bake for 30 minutes, or until the edges and top are golden brown (cover with foil for the last few minutes if it gets too dark on top).

Remove from the oven and let cool for at least 5 minutes, before using a spatula to loosen the cake around the edges and, if possible, along the bottom. Place a plate on top and flip it over to release the cake. Slice and serve.

3 medium (1¾ to 2lb/850–900g total) baking potatoes

2 Tbsp butter

3 heaping Tbsp finely shredded sage

1 medium leek (about 5¼oz/150g), trimmed slightly, halved lengthwise, and thinly sliced

7oz (200g) Brussels sprouts, trimmed, quartered (or halved if using baby sprouts), and steamed until just tender

1 Tbsp whole grain mustard

Sea salt and freshly ground black pepper

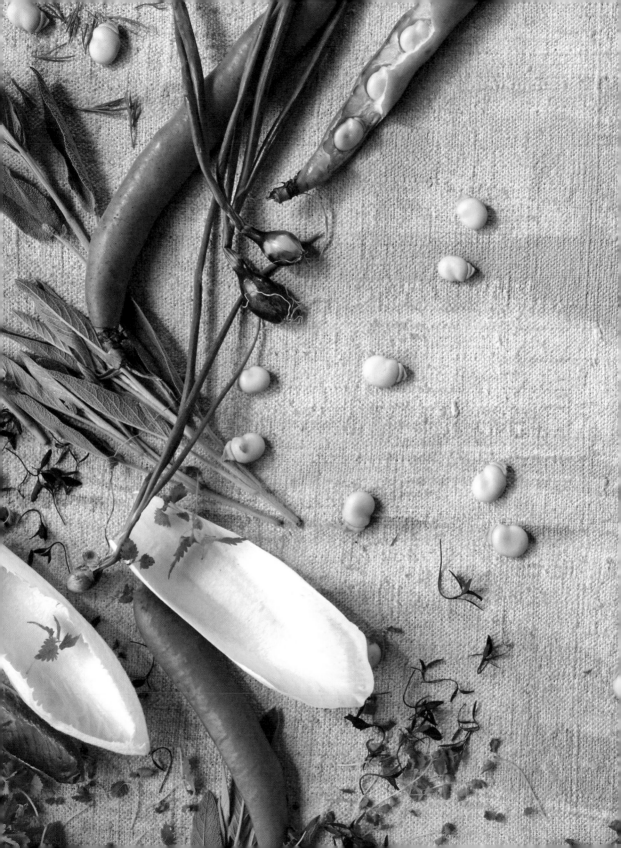

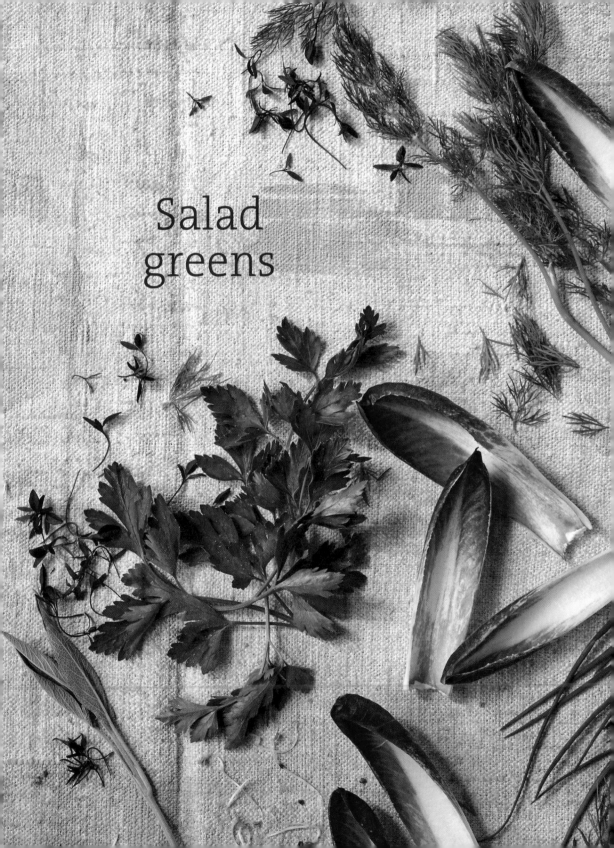

Salad greens

Warm black rice noodle salad

This is a subtle, comforting dish, best served still slightly warm. If you are having this as a main course, add some cooked mung beans or other protein of your choice and perhaps a few halved cherry tomatoes for color. If you cannot find black rice noodles (which provide a great color contrast), regular soba or rice noodles will do just fine. SERVES 4 AS A SIDE DISH

Cook the rice noodles until *al dente*, according to the package directions, then drain, rinse well, and transfer to a large mixing bowl. Toss to coat with a little untoasted sesame or olive oil (to prevent the noodles from sticking together) and a pinch of salt, and set aside.

Heat the canola oil in a pan and fry the shallot with a pinch of salt over medium to high heat for a few minutes or until soft, stirring regularly to avoid burning (some browning is fine).

Add the garlic and five-spice powder and cook for another couple of minutes before adding the bok choy stems. At this point you may want to add some water to deglaze the pan and help the bok choy cook, but make sure you cook the pan dry before adding the leaves.

When the stems are tender, add the leaves and cook until just wilted, for about 30 seconds. Scrape into the bowl with the noodles, then add the remaining salad ingredients to the bowl.

Combine all the dressing ingredients, with salt to taste, in a jar, screw on the lid, and give it a good shake. Taste and adjust the seasoning if necessary—the dressing should taste very intense, as its flavor is diluted once added to the salad. Dress the salad and gently toss to coat.

3oz (80g) black rice noodles

Untoasted (virgin) sesame oil, or extra-virgin olive oil

1 tsp canola oil, or other neutral-tasting cooking oil

1 echalion (banana) shallot, chopped into small dice

2 large garlic cloves, finely chopped

1 tsp Chinese five-spice powder (see page 155 to make your own)

10½oz (300g) bok choy or tatsoi, stalks finely chopped and leaves torn into smaller pieces (or left whole if small)

⅔ cup (100g) double-podded fava beans (see page 66), or peas (fresh or frozen)

1 to 2 scallions, white and green part, finely sliced on the diagonal

3oz (80g/small handful) snow peas, trimmed and any strings removed

1 thin yellow or green zucchini (3 to 3½oz/80 to 100g), finely sliced on the diagonal using a mandolin or vegetable swivel peeler

Sea salt

FOR THE DRESSING

1 Tbsp finely chopped shallot

1 garlic clove, finely chopped

3 Tbsp untoasted (virgin) sesame oil

1½ Tbsp brown (or regular) rice vinegar

½ tsp wasabi powder or paste, or to taste

1 to 1½ Tbsp tamari or shoyu

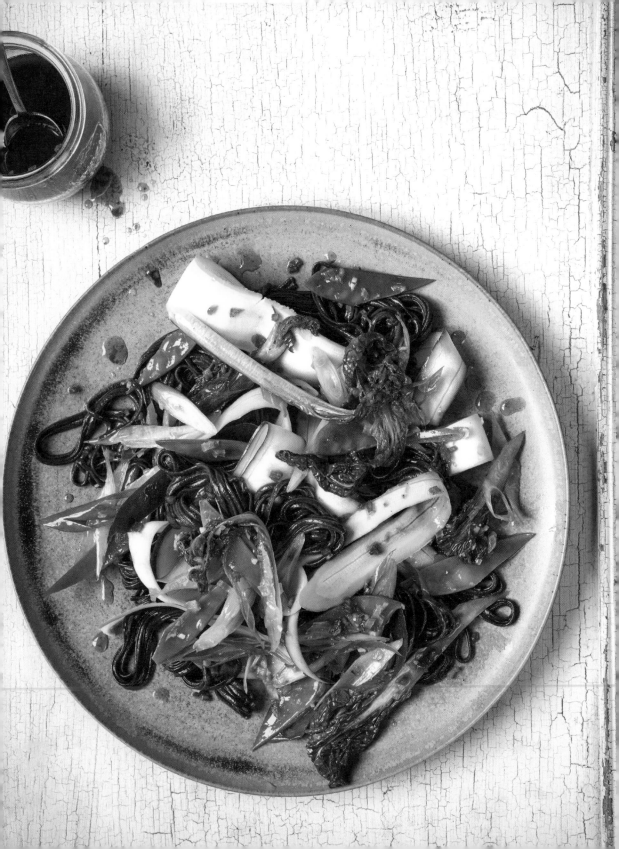

Lettuce cups with sticky brown rice and vegetable crudités

I love meals that invite involvement from diners. It allows them to let their hair down, get their hands dirty, and tailor-make each bite to suit their taste. The dressing and sauce for the rice can be made in advance, and the prepared crudites will keep well for a few hours in an airtight container in the refrigerator. SERVES 4

Combine all the ingredients for the dressing in a small bowl and set aside. Prepare the Sticky Brown Rice following the method on page 156.

While the rice is cooking, put the coconut flesh and water, ginger, garlic, chile, lime zest and juice, oil, fish sauce, and a pinch of salt in a blender, and process to a relatively smooth sauce.

Heat the canola oil in a pan and sauté the scallions with a pinch of salt for a minute or so.

Stir into the sticky rice with the coconut sauce, as soon as the rice is cooked.

Give each guest a head or two of lettuce and a plate, then place the dressing, sticky rice, vegetables, and chicken/tofu in the center of the table and enjoy watching your guests fill each lettuce leaf to their own taste.

FOR THE DRESSING
½ cup (15g/very small handful) cilantro, finely chopped

½ tsp shoyu or tamari

½ tsp fish sauce (optional)

1 Tbsp rice vinegar

½ to 1 Tbsp palm sugar (or dark brown sugar)

1 tsp grated peeled ginger

Juice of 1 lime (1½ to 2 Tbsp)

1 Tbsp untoasted (virgin) sesame oil

1 tsp sesame seeds

FOR THE STICKY RICE
1 quantity of hot Sticky Brown Rice (page 156)

1oz (30g) fresh coconut flesh (the mature meat, sold cubed in grocery stores)

2 Tbsp coconut water, preferably unpasteurized

1 tsp grated peeled ginger

1 medium garlic clove, finely chopped

½ to 1 red Thai chile, finely chopped (seeds and/or membranes removed if you prefer it less spicy)

Grated zest and juice (1 to 1½ Tbsp) of 1 small lime

2 Tbsp avocado oil, or untoasted (virgin) sesame oil

½ to 1 tsp fish sauce, to taste

1 tsp canola oil

4 scallions, thinly sliced, plus extra to serve

Sea salt

TO SERVE
4 or more baby cos or Boston lettuces, trimmed

1 medium carrot, cut into matchsticks

¾ cup (70g) sugar snap peas or snow peas, trimmed, any strings removed, cut into matchsticks

¼ large cucumber, cut into matchsticks

Shredded, cooked chicken, fried tofu, or sliced, cooked beef fillet (optional)

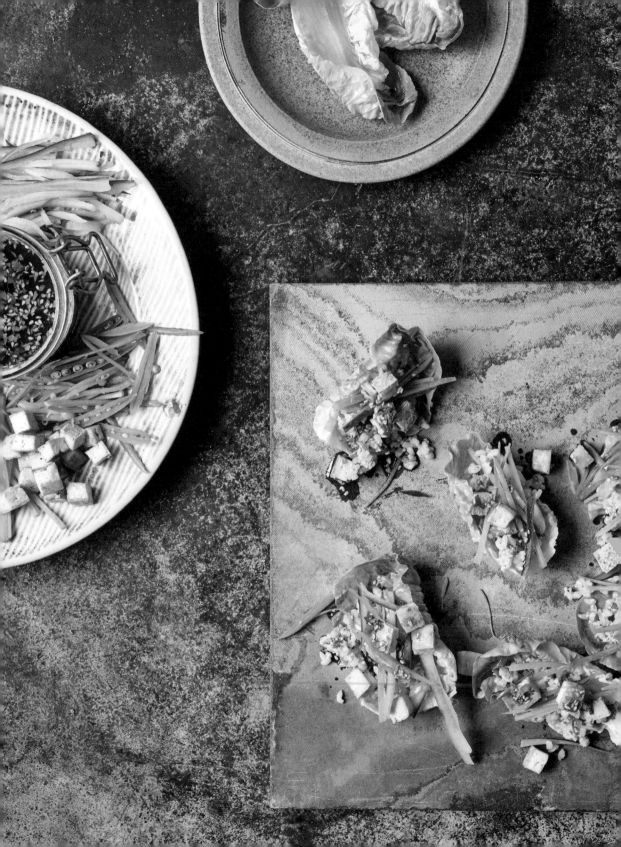

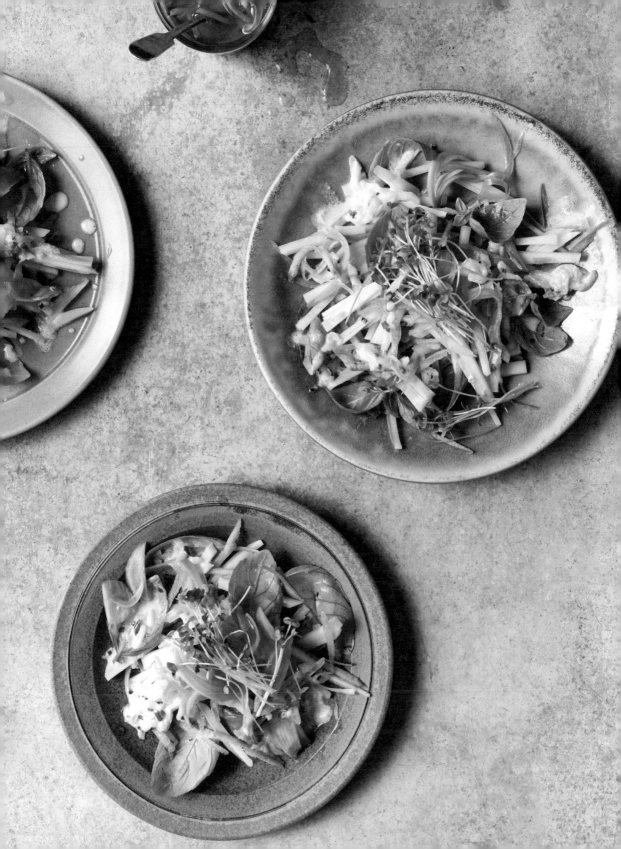

Kohlrabi and pickled onion salad

When all you crave on a bleak, lazy, or stressful day is something crunchy and cheeky, yet deeply satisfying, make this salad. Kohlrabi, either the whitish-green or purple-skinned variety, is not often available at regular grocery stores, but most local and ethnic grocers stock them. Cucumbers are notorious for drawing water, so let it drain for as long as possible and only dress the salad just before serving. SERVES 4 AS A SIDE DISH

For the dressing, mix the grated cucumber with the salt and let drain in a colander set over a plate or bowl.

Mix together the remaining dressing ingredients and set aside.

For the pickled onion, whisk all the ingredients except the onion in a small bowl until the sugar and salt have dissolved. Add the onion slices and ensure everything is covered with the liquid. Set aside for about 1 hour, or until the onion has turned bright pink. Drain, removing the juniper berries.

For the salad, toss the kohlrabi, carrot, basil, and pickled onion with the dressing and arrange on a serving plate. Sprinkle over the cress and tuck in right away.

FOR THE DRESSING

½ medium cucumber, peeled, halved lengthwise, seeded (using an apple corer or teaspoon), and coarsely grated

Large pinch of sea salt

2 Tbsp mayonnaise (see page 154 to make your own, but omit the tarragon)

1 Tbsp lemon juice (about ½ lemon)

2 Tbsp extra-virgin olive oil

Pinch of unrefined brown sugar

1 Tbsp finely chopped chives

FOR THE PICKLED ONION

1 Tbsp coarse sea salt

1 Tbsp unrefined brown sugar

½ cup (125ml) cider vinegar

5 juniper berries, lightly bashed but left whole

5 peppercorns, crushed

1 medium red onion, cut in half through the core, peeled, and thinly sliced

FOR THE SALAD

1 kohlrabi (12¼ to 14oz/350 to 400g), peeled and julienned

1 medium carrot, coarsely grated

Handful of basil leaves, torn into smaller pieces

2 large handfuls of cress

Raw bitters salad

This immensely health-supportive salad is very tasty, as well as being lovely to look at. Most bitter foods are not only very nutrient dense but also help to absorb those nutrients, as they stimulate the production of gastric acid in the stomach. The better your food is digested, the more nutrients you will absorb from your food. Bitters balance your taste buds and control sweet cravings, while also boosting your metabolism and fighting free radicals. Serve with Macadamia Nut Spread (see page 157) when you need a little more substance. SERVES 4 TO 6

1 small radicchio, leaves torn

1¾ to 2½oz (50 to 70g) wild or regular arugula

2 purple or white chicory, leaves torn

1 red grapefruit, peeled and segmented

1 pink grapefruit, peeled and segmented

Large handful of snow peas, trimmed

¾ cup (110g) freshly shelled petits pois or garden peas, or frozen peas blanched in boiling water for 10 seconds and refreshed in ice-cold water

2 large avocados, sliced or diced

½ cup (75g) mixed sunflower and pumpkin seeds

Large handful of basil leaves, finely shredded (see Note on page 40)

FOR THE DRESSING
1 tsp light miso paste, preferably unpasteurized

⅓ cup (80ml) cider vinegar, preferably unpasteurized

½ to 1 Tbsp maple syrup

1 tsp Dijon mustard

1 cup (250ml) extra-virgin olive oil

1 Tbsp finely chopped shallots or red onion

2 cups (50g/1 bunch) parsley, finely chopped

Sea salt and freshly ground black pepper

Toss all the salad ingredients together in a bowl.

For the dressing, whisk together the miso paste, vinegar, maple syrup, mustard, and some salt and pepper. While whisking, add the olive oil in a thin but steady stream, until emulsified. Stir in the shallots and parsley, then toss through the salad.

Rainbow slaw

Every cook should have a good coleslaw recipe in their repertoire. This one is particularly refreshing and tantalizing, and the dressing takes it out of the sphere of the ordinary. SERVES 4 TO 6

½ large pineapple, peeled and "eyes" removed

½ small red cabbage (about 8¾oz/250g), finely shredded

½ napa cabbage (about 8¾ oz/250g), finely shredded

2½ cups (350g) coarsely grated carrots

1 small romaine lettuce head, halved lengthwise and finely shredded

1oz (25g/1 bunch) chives

20 large mint leaves, finely shredded (see Note on page 40)

2 red chiles, very finely chopped

Handful of dry-roasted peanuts (or other nuts)

FOR THE DRESSING
2 tsp shoyu or tamari

2 Tbsp cider vinegar

1 heaped Tbsp grated peeled ginger

1 Tbsp untoasted (virgin) sesame oil

1 Tbsp toasted sesame oil

2 Tbsp unsalted peanut (or other nut) butter

1 tsp raw honey

½ tsp sea salt

For the dressing, put all the ingredients in a glass jar, screw on the lid, and shake vigorously. Set aside.

Grate the pineapple on the coarse side of a box grater. I usually do this on a tray, as it does get messy. Scoop the pineapple flesh into a colander or strainer, set it over a bowl, and let drain.

Put the shredded cabbages, carrots, and lettuce into a large mixing bowl. Snip the bunch of chives into tiny pieces straight into the bowl using scissors. Add the mint and chiles.

Add the drained pineapple to the salad with enough dressing to coat. Give it a good mix and serve with the peanuts sprinkled on top.

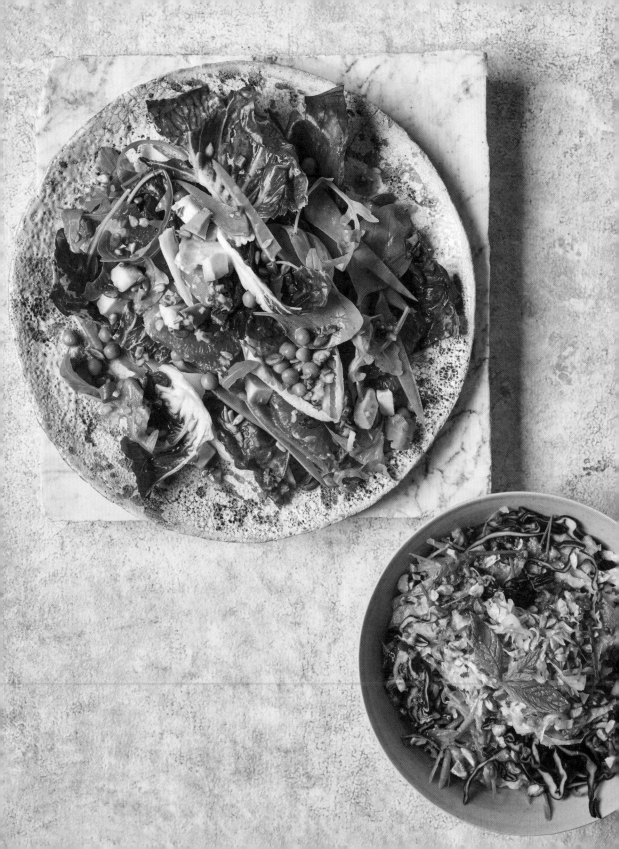

Spiced grain and kale salad

This is a virtuous salad that manages to fill you up and taste great. If you don't have ready-cooked portions of grains and lentils in the freezer (which makes this salad a whole lot easier to prepare), follow the directions in the Note below. Use double quantities of quinoa, instead of the barley, if you are avoiding gluten. And feel free to use whole spices and grind them yourself. SERVES 4

Heat the butter in a medium pan, add the onions, and sauté over gentle heat until they start to soften. Increase the heat to medium and cook, stirring regularly, until they start to caramelize, for about 30 minutes.

Meanwhile, put the kale into a big mixing bowl, add the salt, lemon juice, and olive oil, then massage the leaves with your fingertips for a few minutes, until they become soft and silky. Add the remaining salad ingredients and set aside.

For the dressing, toast the spices in a dry frying pan over medium heat until they become fragrant. Transfer to a jar with the rest of the dressing ingredients, with salt and pepper to taste, screw the lid on tightly, and give a vigorous shake. Pour the dressing over the salad and toss to coat.

NOTE:
To cook the grains and lentils from scratch, soak about 45g each of the quinoa, barley, basmati rice, and lentils separately in plenty of water overnight, then rinse each separately and start by bringing the barley and a large pinch of salt to a boil in four times its volume of fresh water. After 10 minutes (or 20 if you are using pot barley), add the lentils and rice, and after another 15 minutes or so, the quinoa. Cook for another 5 to 10 minutes or until all the grains and lentils are tender, then remove from the heat. Strain off any water, return the mixture to the pan and cover with a lid for another 5 minutes.

1½ Tbsp butter

2 large onions, cut in half through the core, peeled, and sliced

3½oz (100g) kale, tough stalks removed, chopped

Pinch of sea salt

½ Tbsp lemon juice

½ Tbsp extra-virgin olive oil

Generous 2 cups (400g) mixture of cooked quinoa, pearl (or pot) barley, brown basmati rice, and Puy lentils

¼ cup (35g) raisins and/or dried cherries

½ cup (70g) shelled, unroasted hazelnuts, roughly chopped

¾ cup (20g/1 small bunch) dill, largest stalks removed, finely chopped

FOR THE DRESSING
¼ tsp ground cloves

½ tsp freshly grated nutmeg

1½ tsp ground cumin

1½ tsp ground coriander

1½ tsp ground fennel seeds

2 Tbsp extra-virgin olive oil

Grated zest of 1 lemon

⅓ to ½ cup (80 to 125ml) kefir or stirred plain yogurt

1 to 2 tsp sea salt

Freshly ground black pepper

Sea vegetable salad

This is a great salad to introduce people to sea vegetables. The mix of sea vegetables can include arame (with a mild sweetness and chewy texture), hijiki (bolder and with a subtle anise flavor), and dulse (with an earthy taste). All sea veg need to be rehydrated by soaking in room-temperature water just until pliable (10 minutes for arame and dulse, 20 minutes for hiziki), then drained and squeezed. Most grocery stores (and healthfood stores) sell sea veg in the Asian sections. SERVES 4 (OR 6 AS A SIDE DISH)

Handful of mixed sea vegetables, rehydrated according to the package directions, and finely chopped if large

2 medium red and/or golden beet, peeled and cut into matchsticks

1 watermelon radish (about 4½ oz/130g), cut into matchsticks

2 celery stalks, cut into thirds and then into matchsticks

1 large cucumber (11¾ to 12¼oz/330 to 350g), peeled, halved lengthwise, seeded (use an apple corer or teaspoon), and sliced into thin half-moons

1⅔ cups (250g) seedless red grapes, halved

Few handfuls of shredded red or white chicory, baby arugula, or lamb's lettuce (mâche) (optional)

FOR THE DRESSING
2 Tbsp lemon juice (about 1 small lemon)

1 medium garlic clove, peeled

1½ tsp honey

⅓ cup (80ml) extra-virgin olive oil

2½ Tbsp light miso paste

1 heaping tsp grated peeled ginger

2 thin scallions, or 1 thick, green part thinly sliced and set aside for the salad, white part roughly chopped

For the dressing, blend all the ingredients, except the scallion slices, in a blender until creamy.

Combine the salad ingredients, including the scallions, and toss with enough dressing to coat.

Serve with the Watercress Oat Cakes (page 136) and the Smoked Mackerel and Watercress Mousse (page 52), or warm falafels.

PHOTOGRAPH ON PAGE 53

Lamb's lettuce, pumpkin seed, and apple salad

This is definitely a green salad, with the soft and silky lamb's lettuce, crunchy Boston lettuce, and sweet-sour apples. The pumpkin seed oil does add a lovely flavor, and is a fantastic ingredient to have in your pantry, but feel free to use avocado oil or just olive oil instead. You will most likely have some leftover dressing, but it keeps well in the refrigerator for a few days and can be enjoyed with any salad or shredded vegetables. If you are preparing the salad in advance, do not dress it until just before serving and toss the apple slices in some lemon juice diluted with water to prevent browning. SERVES 4 TO 6

3½oz (100g) lamb's lettuce (mâche)

2 Boston lettuces, leaves separated

2 green apples, cored, halved and sliced

1½ cups (150g) sugar snap peas, any strings removed

½ cup (80g) pumpkin seeds, toasted in a dry frying pan until they start to pop

FOR THE DRESSING
1 small or ½ large ripe avocado

⅓ cup (80ml) lemon juice (2 to 3 lemons)

1 to 1½ Tbsp maple syrup or honey, to taste

½ cup (125ml) mixture of pumpkin seed oil and olive oil (1:3 ratio), or all olive oil

1 tsp Dijon mustard

1oz (30g/small handful) fresh cilantro, thickest stems removed

Put all the salad ingredients, except the pumpkin seeds, into a large bowl.

In a blender, blend together the ingredients for the dressing and pour enough over the salad to coat lightly and evenly, when gently tossed.

Sprinkle with the toasted pumpkin seeds and serve immediately.

Herb salad

This is a wonderfully refreshing green salad that is delicious with a rich or heavy main course, or served as a first course to awaken the palate. I sometimes add a finely shredded chicory or a tomato. Use up all the dressing—the salad needs it. If you don't like the sharp taste of raw onion, soak it in cold water for 15 minutes after chopping, then drain. SERVES 4

1 to 2 pita breads, cut into very thin strips

1 head romaine lettuce, coarsely chopped

1 to generous 1 cup (25 to 30g/1 small bunch) flat-leaf parsley, leaves only, finely chopped

3 to 4 sprigs (15g) basil, leaves only, torn into bite-size pieces

⅓ cup (10g/½ small bunch) dill, thickest part of stalks discarded, roughly chopped

½ cup (15g/½ bunch) chives, snipped into small pieces

2 to 3 mint sprigs, leaves only, finely shredded

⅓ cup (10g/1 handful) tarragon sprigs, leaves only, roughly chopped

FOR THE DRESSING
1 Tbsp finely chopped red onion

½ tsp dried oregano

1 Tbsp finely chopped fresh thyme leaves

3 to 4 oregano sprigs, leaves only (about 2 heaping Tbsp), finely chopped (or use a little more dried if you can't find fresh)

1 Tbsp red wine vinegar

3 Tbsp extra-virgin olive oil

Large pinch of unrefined brown sugar

Large pinch of sea salt

Preheat the oven to 350°F (180°C).

Spread the strips of pita out on a baking sheet in a single layer and bake in the oven for 20 to 25 minutes until crunchy.

For the dressing, put all the ingredients in a glass jar, screw the lid on tightly, and shake vigorously until the sugar has dissolved.

Toss the salad ingredients and pita chips together. Dress the salad and serve immediately.

Lentil and spinach salad

Hearty, moreish, and a staple on my weekly menu, the secret to this dish is a delicious aged balsamic vinegar and lovely ripe avocados. Add a cup of cooked brown rice to turn it into a filling lunch option. Make a batch of the slow-roasted tomatoes and enjoy them on toast, with scrambled eggs or blended into soups and sauces throughout the week. SERVES 2 TO 4

5¼oz (150g) baby leaf spinach

1¾ cups (350g) cooked black (or "beluga") or Puy lentils (see page 152)

1⅓ cups (150g) crumbled goat milk feta cheese

4 to 5 artichoke hearts (about 2¼oz/60g) in oil, drained and quartered

3 scallions, green and white part, trimmed and thinly sliced

3½ to 4¼oz (100 to 125g) Slow-Roasted Cherry Tomatoes (page 154)

2 ripe avocados, cut into medium dice

FOR THE DRESSING
½ Tbsp aged balsamic vinegar

½ tsp Dijon mustard

½ tsp honey or maple syrup, to taste

¼ cup (60ml) extra-virgin olive oil

Sea salt and freshly ground black pepper

Toss all the salad ingredients together, setting aside some feta and scallion slices to garnish.

For the dressing, put all the ingredients, with salt and pepper to taste, in a jar, screw on the lid, and shake vigorously until emulsified. Dress the salad and toss gently just before serving.

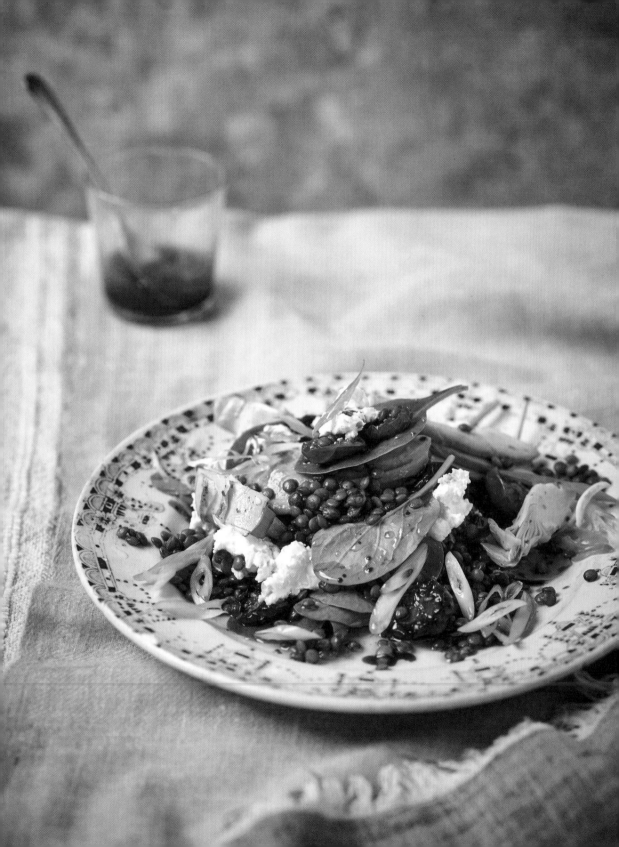

The love salad

So-called because it's perfect for a romantic, celebratory dinner, this salad is a satisfying meal and quite beautiful to look at. You do need to start on it the night before, though, as both the cheese and duck need some time. Omit the duck if you prefer a vegetarian salad. SERVES 4

Score the duck skin in a crisscross pattern using a very sharp knife, being careful not to cut into the meat. Whisk the balsamic vinegar, honey, oil, and lemon juice together in a bowl large enough to fit the duck snugly, then add the garlic and rosemary. Add the duck breasts to the marinade, coating them well, then marinate, skin side up, in the refrigerator for at least 12 hours.

For the salad, line a strainer with cheesecloth and scoop the yogurt into the center. Place the strainer in a bowl, cover with a clean dishtowel, and let strain in the refrigerator overnight.

The next day, preheat the oven to 320°F/160°C. Cut the beet into thin slices, 2mm thick, using a mandolin, and set aside any offcuts in a small bowl. Toss the beet slices with the olive oil and a little salt, transfer to a baking sheet, and bake for 35 to 45 minutes, removing any slices that have browned sooner, as they will taste bitter if too dark. Set aside to cool and turn crisp.

While the beet is roasting, remove the duck breast from the marinade, reserving the marinade, pat them dry, and place skin side down in a heavy, preferably cast-iron, frying pan. Cook over low to medium heat for 10 to 12 minutes, until the skin is crisp and brown. Do not try to rush this step, as the low temperature will help render the fat in the skin. Turn the duck over and cook for another 2 minutes, then remove from the pan.

Use paper towels to wipe the pan clean, turn the heat up to high, return the duck to the pan skin side up, and pour in the reserved marinade. Simmer for less than a minute, to reduce the marinade, then remove the pan from the heat, cover, and keep warm for at least 10 minutes. The residual heat will finish cooking the duck.

While the duck is resting, scoop the goat curd from the cheesecloth-lined strainer and transfer to a bowl. Season with salt and pepper and stir in just enough of the beet juice that will have collected in the bowl of offcuts to color the cheese a lovely pink.

For the dressing, put all the ingredients in a glass jar, screw the lid on tightly, and shake until the honey has dissolved.

Put the greens, berries, and radishes in a dish. Slice the duck breasts and add, along with the dressing, then toss to coat. Pile the beet slices on top and dollop the fresh curd to the side.

2 duck breasts, skin on

3 Tbsp balsamic vinegar

1 Tbsp honey

3 Tbsp extra-virgin olive oil

Juice of ½ lemon

2 large garlic cloves, peeled and bashed with the flat side of a large knife

2 rosemary sprigs

FOR THE SALAD
Scant 1 cup (200g) full-cream thick goat milk yogurt

1lb 2oz (500g) raw beet, peeled

1½ Tbsp extra-virgin olive oil

1¾ cups (100g) mixture of beet greens (finely shredded if not young and tender), radish greens, and baby ruby chard

1⅓ cups (200g) strawberries

Scant 1 cup (100g) raspberries

5 large red and/or purple radishes, very thinly sliced using a mandolin

Sea salt and freshly ground black pepper

FOR THE DRESSING
3 Tbsp extra-virgin olive oil

1 Tbsp raspberry vinegar (or crush a few raspberries and mix with 1 Tbsp apple cider vinegar)

1 tsp honey

1 tsp each of black and white poppy seeds (or black only, if white is hard to find)

¼ tsp cayenne pepper

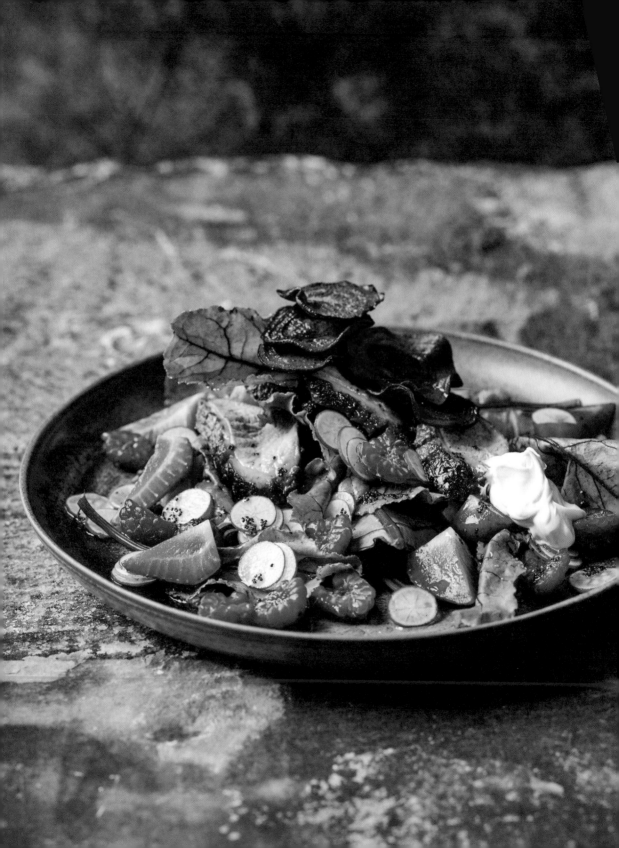

The super salad

The term "superfood" has lost its gloss, having been overused by gym bunnies and abused by marketeers in the food industry. But some foods are most definitely big hitters in the nutrient department and are the opposite of empty calories. Here is a salad that makes use of some of these delicious, naturally potent foods that leave you feeling nourished, not duped. Soaking the quinoa overnight prior to cooking will improve its nutritional value and make it more digestible. SERVES 4

Preheat the oven to 320°F (160°C).

Wash the broccoli and dry well by shaking off any excess water. Trim, but leave some of the stem intact, then separate into similar-size florets, cutting through the stem lengthwise to give each floret a little handle.

Toss the broccoli with the oil and a little salt, spread out on a baking sheet, and roast in the oven for 20 to 25 minutes, or until just tender, with a delicious crunch and caramelized around the edges. Do not let it get too dark, or it will taste bitter.

If you prefer toasted nuts, toast the walnuts on a baking sheet in the oven at the same time as you are roasting the broccoli, for about 10 to 15 minutes, or until crunchy. Let cool, then roughly chop. If not toasting, just roughly chop.

For the dressing, put all the ingredients in a glass jar, screw the lid on tightly, and give it a good shake.

Toss all the ingredients for the salad together, except the hemp seeds. Add the dressing, toss to coat and sprinkle over the hemp seeds to serve.

NOTE:
An easy way to remove the pomegranate seeds is to cut the fruit in half then, holding one half over a large bowl with the cut side facing down, knock the tough outer peel with the back of a large metal spoon until the seeds pop out.

12¼oz (350g/2 small to medium heads) broccoli

1 to 2 Tbsp chili oil or regular olive oil

Scant ⅔ cup (60g) shelled, unroasted walnuts

Large handful of salad sprouts of your choice (sunflower seed sprouts are particularly good, but mung bean or alfalfa sprouts work too)

1 cup (200g) cooked quinoa (¾ cup/ 115g dried)

Seeds of 1 pomegranate (see Note below)

1⅓cups (180g) cooked red kidney beans (see page 152)

1 bunch (about 100g) watercress, snipped into smaller pieces using scissors

2 Tbsp shelled hemp seeds and/or sunflower seeds

Sea salt

FOR THE DRESSING
1 Tbsp tahini (sesame seed paste— preferably not the raw or unroasted kind)

½ cup (125ml) extra-virgin olive oil

2 Tbsp lemon juice (about 1 lemon)

2 tsp honey or maple syrup

2 to 3 tsp freshly grated peeled ginger

1 Tbsp cider vinegar

Small handful of parsley, leaves only, finely chopped

Small handful of cilantro, thickest stalks removed, finely chopped

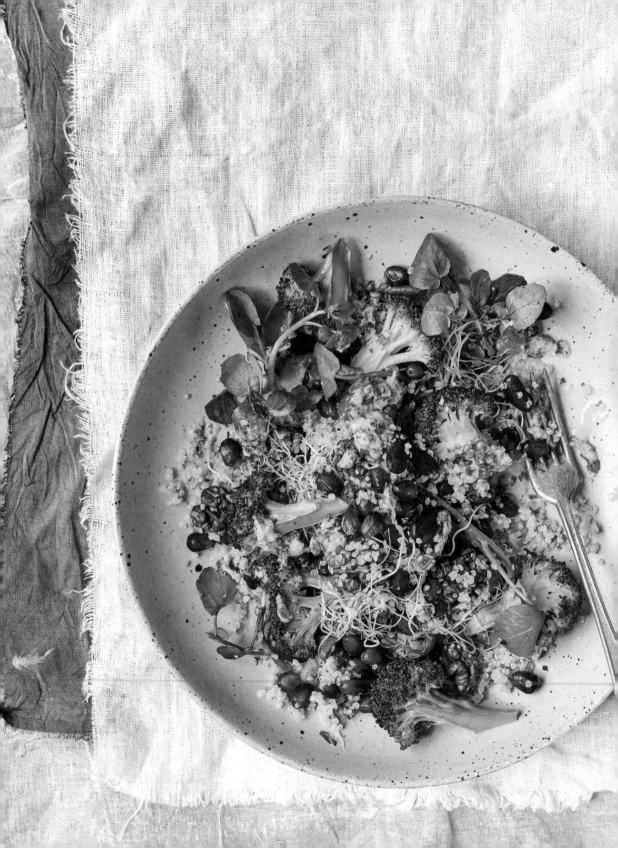

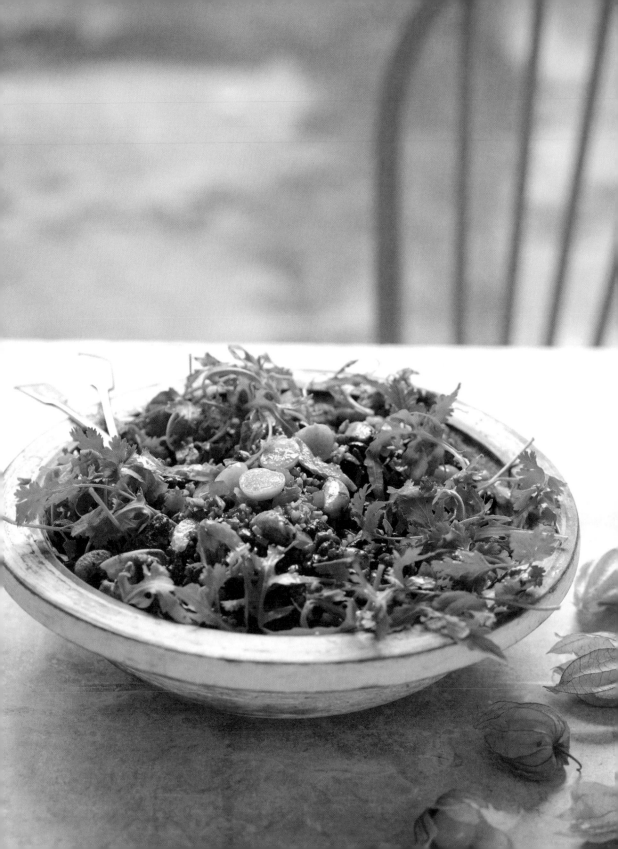

Mexican rice and black bean salad

This is one for the adults, but you can certainly use some of the components to put together a salad for the little ones too. The physalis (also known as cape gooseberry) is the superhero of the berry world. Closely related to the tomato and native to countries in Latin America, they are a good source of vitamin C, beta-carotene, iron, calcium, and trace amounts of B vitamins. Physalis and fruits of the same family, tomatillos and Chinese lanterns, contain 18 kinds of amino acids and all eight essential amino acids. Although red rice is not a typical Mexican ingredient, it adds a lovely texture and flavor to this dish. SERVES 4

For the dressing, combine all the ingredients except the lime zest (set aside for serving) in a glass jar, screw on the lid, and shake vigorously until it is well mixed and emulsified.

For the salad, put all the ingredients except the arugula in a mixing bowl and give them a good stir. Mix in the arugula and, just before serving, pour over the dressing to taste. If you have any left over, it will keep well in the refrigerator for up to a week and is particularly good with mashed avocado and baked potatoes.

To serve, roughly chop the Roasted Spiced Nuts and sprinkle over the salad with the reserved lime zest.

NOTE:
The rice and beans (see page 152 for cooking directions), the Roasted Spiced Nuts, and the dressing can be cooked and prepared at least a couple of days in advance, as long as you keep the rice and beans refrigerated and the nuts in an airtight container. If you choose to use canned beans, bear in mind that they are almost always softer and mushier than cooked dry beans, so consider refrying them before adding to the salad, to add some texture.

⅓ to ½ quantity of Roasted Spiced Nuts (page 156)

FOR THE DRESSING
Grated zest and juice (1½ Tbsp) of 1 lime

½ Tbsp almond (or peanut) butter

½ to 1 tsp honey, to taste

Large pinch of sea salt

¼ cup (60ml) extra-virgin olive oil

2 tsp finely chopped oregano leaves (or 1 tsp dried)

1 to 2 heaping tsp finely chopped jalapeño (about ½ to 1 chile), seeds left in

FOR THE SALAD
1¼ cups (150g) cooked red Camargue rice (⅓ cup/65g uncooked)

1¼ cups (180g) cooked black beans (just tender and not mushy) (⅓ cup/60g uncooked, see page 152)

1 red bell pepper, core and seeds removed, diced

2 handfuls of physalis (cape gooseberries), decaped and halved

2 celery stalks, thinly sliced on the diagonal

1 to 2 cups (25 to 50g/1 to 2 small bunches) cilantro, large stalks removed, finely chopped

1¾ to 2½oz (50 to 70g) arugula leaves

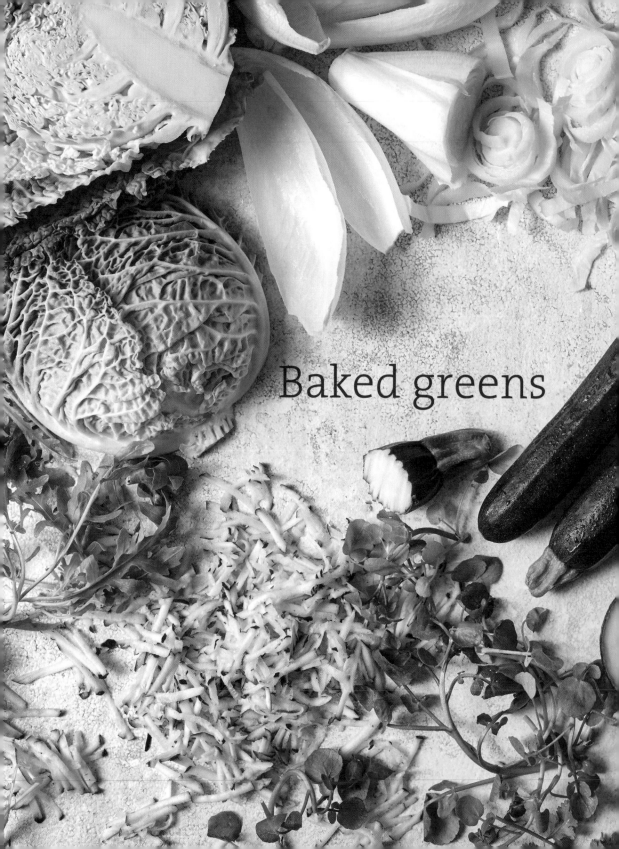

Baked greens

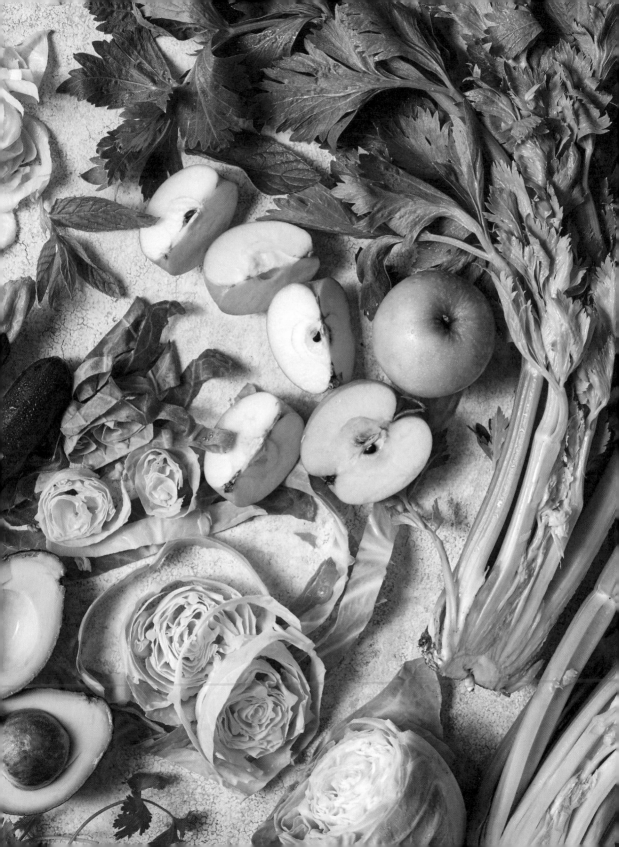

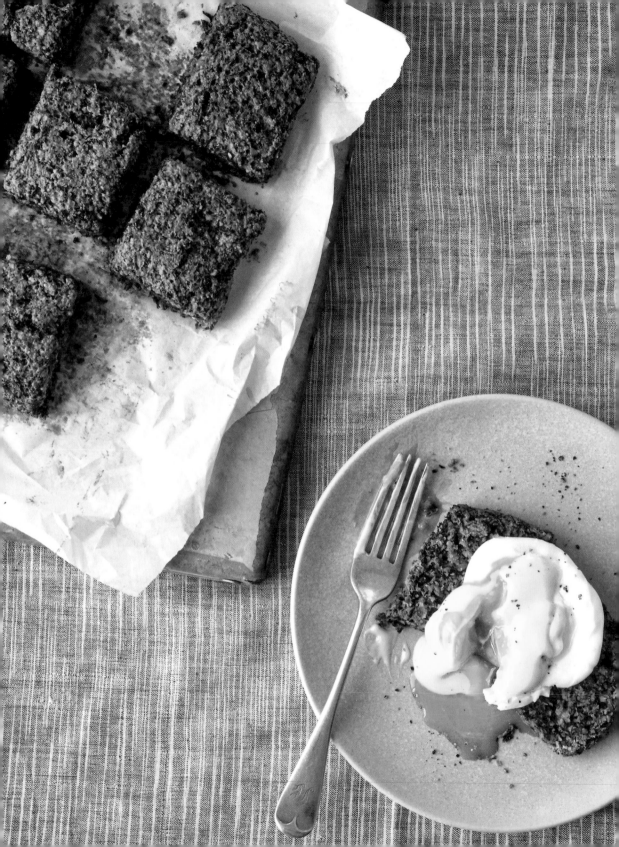

Oat and kale breakfast biscuits

Always on the look-out for interesting meals to start the day with, I regularly make this for my family and friends. Nutritious, filling, and different yet familiar, it ticks all the boxes for a special breakfast dish. Being gluten-free, it is a very crumbly biscuit, but no less delicious for it. Instead of the kale and nutmeg, you could add lots of finely chopped chives and cayenne pepper, or a little goat cheese and chopped thyme leaves. Roughly chopped black olives and finely chopped rosemary make a good addition, too. MAKES 9 SMALLISH BISCUITS

Preheat the oven to 350°F (180°C) and line a medium baking sheet with baking parchment.

Heat the olive oil in a pan, add the onion, and sweat over gentle heat until soft and translucent. Add the kale and sauté until tender and cooked, then process in a food processor, or chop very finely by hand, press out any moisture and set aside to cool completely.

Spoon half the oat flakes into the food processor (no need to rinse) and blitz until very fine. Add the rest of the flakes and pulse a few times until the larger flakes are broken down slightly. Add the baking powder, baking soda, nutmeg, and salt, and pulse to mix.

Add the cubed butter or coconut oil and pulse until the mixture resembles wet sand. Add the cooled kale and onion mixture, the chia seed gel, apple puree, and egg, and process until the mixtures comes together. It should be a little on the sticky side.

Using a spatula, scrape the dough out onto the lined baking sheet. Form into a square about ¾in (2cm) thick, then score into 9 smaller squares, leaving them joined together. Bake in the oven for 20 to 25 minutes until golden, rotating the sheet halfway through cooking.

Carefully slide a spatula under the biscuits to loosen them from the baking parchment, then separate the pieces using a knife, move them apart a little to give them some room and return to the oven for another 10 to 12 minutes, to crisp the edges.

Remove from the oven and cool on a wire rack. Serve with butter, hollandaise, and poached eggs for breakfast.

A little olive oil

1 small onion, diced

3½ oz (100g) kale, stalks removed, roughly chopped

2 cups (200g) oat flakes (certified gluten-free if you are sensitive)

1 tsp baking powder

½ tsp baking soda

½ tsp freshly grated nutmeg

Large pinch of sea salt

1 Tbsp chia seeds, mixed with 2 Tbsp water and stirred until a thick gel forms

½ cup (60g) cold butter (or firm coconut oil, hardened in the refrigerator), cut into small cubes

¼ cup (60ml) apple puree or applesauce (see Introduction on page 143)

1 egg, lightly whisked

Belgian endive and shallot tarte Tatin

This dish is in honor of a tiny little village restaurant in the heart of Burgundy where I was served something similar but, due to severe language barriers, I never found out more than that they had used fresh orange juice. Braising endive in orange juice is quite commonplace in both Britain and France and helps mellow the bitterness. Finish with creamy goat cheese crumbled on top and a drizzle of honey, if serving as a cheese course or dessert. SERVES 4 TO 6

For the pie dough, put the flour, salt, and mustard powder in a food processor and pulse to mix. Add the butter cubes and pulse to the size of very small peas. Add the egg, thyme, and cheese and pulse until the mixture comes together. Scrape into a bowl and knead gently a few times to form a dough. Alternatively, make the dough by hand, by rubbing the butter into the flour, salt, and mustard mixture with your fingertips until it resembles coarse sand, then adding the rest of the ingredients and briefly kneading until it forms a dough.

Flatten the dough into a disk on the counter and roll out, between two large pieces of baking parchment, to a circle that will just fit into a 12-in (30-cm) ovenproof frying pan or Tatin dish. Refrigerate for about 1 hour, until thoroughly chilled and firm.

Preheat the oven to 350°F (180°C).

For the topping, melt the butter in the ovenproof frying pan or Tatin dish. Add the endive, cut sides down, and cook over moderately high heat for about 5 minutes, until sizzling. Put the halved shallots into any gaps you can find (it doesn't matter if they don't lie flat), cover the pan, and bake for 20 minutes.

Turn the endive cut sides up and season with salt and pepper. There should be some lovely caramelization and enough room now for the shallots to lie flat between the endive. Sprinkle over most of the thyme leaves and pour over the orange juice and bake, uncovered, for another 10 minutes. The endive and shallots should be very tender. Turn the endive and shallots cut side down again and set aside in the pan to cool completely.

Increase the oven temperature to 425°F (220°C).

Remove the dough from the refrigerator and warm up for 5 minutes to make it more pliable. Drape it over the cooled vegetables in the pan and bake in the oven for 30 to 35 minutes, until the pastry is crisp and golden.

Using oven mitts to protect your hands, set a large plate upside down on top of the pan, then carefully invert the tart onto the plate. Let cool slightly, then sprinkle over the remaining thyme leaves and cut into wedges. Serve warm with crumbled goat cheese on top.

FOR THE PIE DOUGH

1¾ cups (250g) wholewheat spelt flour

Pinch of sea salt

½ tsp mustard powder

9 Tbsp cold butter, cut into small cubes

1 egg, lightly beaten

1 tsp dried thyme

¼ cup (30g) finely grated Gruyère cheese

FOR THE TOPPING

3 Tbsp butter

3 heads of Belgian endive (about 1lb 2oz/500g), halved lengthwise

10½oz (300g) echalion (banana) shallots, peeled and halved lengthwise

5 thyme sprigs, leaves only

⅓ cup (80ml) fresh orange juice (about 2 medium oranges)

Sea salt and freshly ground black pepper

Crumbled goat cheese, to serve

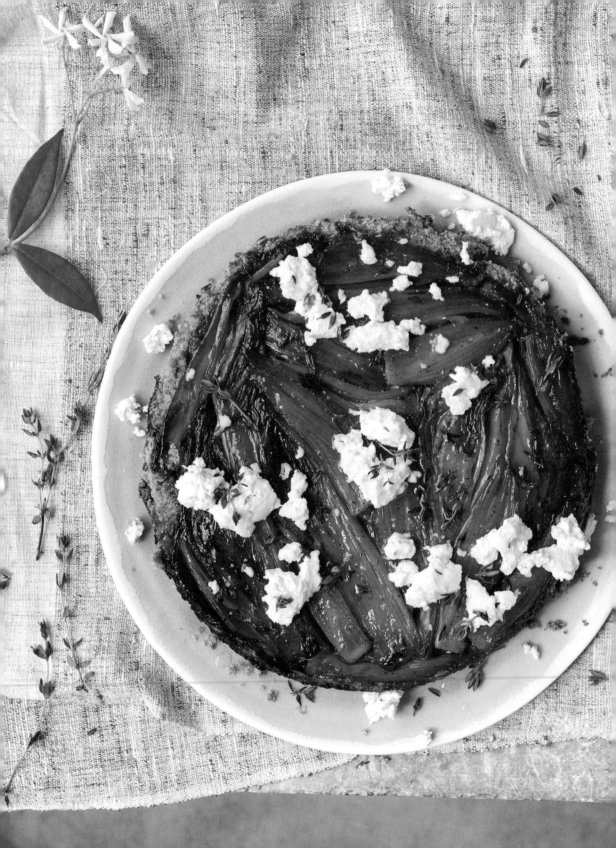

Salmon and samphire tartlets

These posh little quiches are perfect for a special lunch alongside a couple of salads, but also make a good start to an elegant dinner. Substitute the salmon with briefly steamed asparagus pieces if you would like to make a vegetarian version. Or use asparagus if you cannot find samphire (sea beans). This dish really benefits from being baked in deep tart shells, as the shallower versions leave you with too much pastry, too little filling, and easily overcooked fish. MAKES 4 DEEP, 3- TO 3½-IN (8- TO 9-CM) TARTLETS

Grease 4 loose-bottomed, 3- to 3½-in (8- to 9-cm) tart pans, by dipping a pastry brush in oil and brushing the insides.

Put the butter, flour, chervil, and salt in a food processor and blitz until the mixture resembles coarse sand. With the motor running, add the cold water until the dough just starts to come together. Tip out and knead briefly until you have a cohesive, smooth ball of dough.

Roll out the dough thinly between two sheets of wax paper, then cut out 4 circles large enough to line the tart shells (use a large round pastry cutter or lid of a food container). Carefully press each into a tart pan and refrigerate for about 30 minutes, until firm. Meanwhile, preheat the oven to 350°F (180°C).

Bake the tart shells blind (without the filling or any need for pie weights) for 10 to 15 minutes and remove from the oven. Use a pastry brush to brush some of the beaten eggs onto any cracks that may have formed in the tart shells during baking and return them to the oven for another couple of minutes before removing and setting aside to cool slightly.

Meanwhile, place the salmon on a small baking sheet and bake in the oven for no more than 5 minutes (or less if it is a very thin fillet). Remove and use a fork to gently separate the flesh (that will still be mostly raw) from the skin. Set aside.

Heat the oil, butter, or ghee in a small pan and sweat the leek until tender. Let cool before using a blender or stick blender to blend it with the eggs and cream (or milk) until smooth. Stir in the lemon zest, juice, and mustard.

Divide the samphire and flaked salmon between the pastry shells, pour over the egg-and-leek mixture, and bake for 20 minutes, or until set. Let cool for a few minutes before serving, topped with a grinding of black pepper and some finely chopped parsley.

FOR THE PIE DOUGH
Oil, for greasing

2 Tbsp cold butter, cut into small dice

⅔ cup (90g) wholewheat spelt flour, plus extra for dusting

1 heaping tsp dried chervil

Very small pinch of sea salt

1 to 2 Tbsp ice-cold water

FOR THE FILLING
2 eggs, lightly beaten

1 small salmon fillet (about 4½oz/130g), preferably wild

A little coconut oil, butter or ghee

1 small leek (about 5¼oz/150g), trimmed, halved lengthwise, and thinly sliced

3 Tbsp cream, full-cream milk or milk substitute

Grated zest of 1 lemon and 1½ Tbsp juice

1 to 2 tsp whole grain mustard

1 oz (25g) samphire, roughly chopped

TO SERVE
Freshly ground black pepper

Handful of flat-leaf parsley, leaves finely chopped

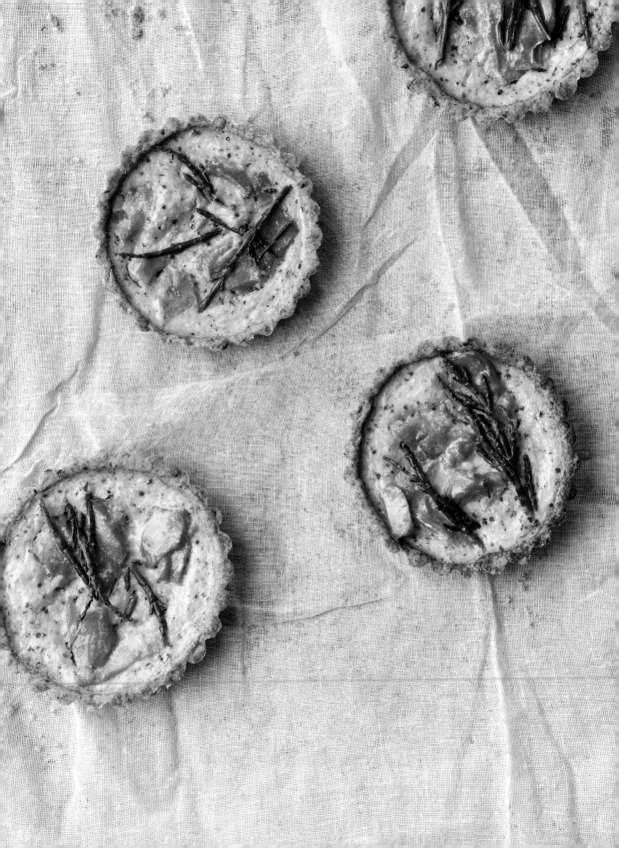

Nori amaranth crackers

Amaranth is naturally gluten-free, very nutritious, and a protein powerhouse. You should be able to find amaranth flour in healthfood stores, or make your own by blitzing about 1 cup amaranth seeds until pulverized in a high-speed blender or spice grinder. The nori can be substituted for a few Tbsp of chopped cilantro, if you prefer.
MAKES 40 TO 50

Scant 1 cup (180g) amaranth flour

½ cup (50g) ground sunflower seeds (use a mini food processor or a spice grinder and be careful not to overprocess)

1 cup (140g) arrowroot powder

½ cup (70g) sesame seeds (ideally black)

2 tsp baking powder

1 tsp fine sea salt

½ tsp freshly cracked black pepper

2 sheets of nori, torn into very little pieces (see Introduction above)

6 Tbsp untoasted (virgin) sesame oil, or olive oil

Scant ½ to ½ cup (100 to 125ml) water

2 Tbsp tamari or shoyu

Preheat the oven to 350°F (180°C).

In a bowl, whisk together the dry ingredients, including the nori, then pour in the oil, most of the water (setting aside a Tbsp or two), and the tamari or shoyu. Mix together, then tip out onto the counter and knead into a malleable dough, adding more water if it seems too dry, but without letting the dough get sticky.

Divide the dough in half and roll each out to about ⅛in (3mm) between two sheets of baking parchment. Remove the top piece of baking parchment and, using a large, sharp knife, cut each dough sheet into about 20 squares or rectangles. Slide the baking parchment onto baking sheets and bake the crackers for 15 to 20 minutes, or until golden and crispy, rotating the sheets once.

Carefully transfer the crackers to a wire rack to cool completely, then break along the cut lines. They keep well for several weeks in an airtight container.

PHOTOGRAPH ON PAGE 51

Watercress oat cakes

The perfect cookie for salmon pâté or Smoked Mackerel and Watercress Mousse (page 52), these are deliciously crumbly with a hint of fennel and a spicy aftertaste from the watercress. The uncooked dough will keep in the refrigerator for several days or can be tightly wrapped in plastic wrap and frozen. I usually bake one log and freeze the other for later use. MAKES 20 TO 40, DEPENDING ON THE LENGTH OF THE LOGS

3½oz (100g) watercress, leaves and stalks

Scant ¾ cup (100g) wholewheat spelt flour

2 cups (200g) medium oatmeal (stoneground groats, not oat flakes or pinhead oats)

1 Tbsp fennel seeds, toasted in a dry frying pan until fragrant (be careful not to burn them)

1½ tsp baking powder

7 Tbsp cold, unsalted butter, cubed (or cold coconut oil, cubed)

Sea salt and freshly ground black pepper

Blitz the watercress in a food processor until finely chopped. Add the flour, oatmeal, toasted fennel seeds, a large pinch of salt, a small pinch of pepper, and the baking powder, and pulse to mix.

Add the cubed butter or coconut oil and process until the mixture comes together. Tip out onto the counter and briefly knead. If it is too crumbly, knead in ice-cold water ½ tsp at a time, until the dough becomes malleable.

Divide the dough in half and form two rectangular logs (I use the flat side of my large chef's knife to get the sides smooth). Loosely cover with plastic wrap and chill for 1 hour, or until completely firm.

Preheat the oven to 350°F (180°C) and line two baking sheets with baking parchment.

Remove one log from the refrigerator and slice into cookies about ¼in (5mm) thick. Arrange on the baking sheets, leaving some space between each. Repeat with the other log. Bake for 25 minutes, until the cakes are golden and browning around the edges. Let cool on the baking sheets. They keep well for several weeks, stored in an airtight container.

PHOTOGRAPH ON PAGE 52

Chard and feta savory muffins

These muffins (not the eggs-Benedict-kind, but the American-baked-goods-kind) are great to take along to a picnic or as an after-school snack. Look for traditionally made, soft cooking chorizo that has no added nasties, and choose the mild version if you are feeding youngsters. If you are vegetarian, leave out the chorizo and fry the onion and chard in a little butter or coconut oil, but add another tsp of smoked paprika powder and perhaps a little more cayenne pepper. MAKES 12

Sauté the chorizo in a hot, dry frying pan until the fat starts to render, then add the onion and cook until soft and translucent. Scrape the mixture into a bowl.

Add the chard stalks to the pan with a small pinch of salt. Cook until tender, for 5 to 10 minutes, depending on size. If they are drying out, add a splash or three of water to the pan. Add the chard leaves and cook for about a minute, or until wilted.

Tip all the chard into a food processor or onto a cutting board, and chop finely. Add this to the chorizo and onion mix, then set aside to cool.

Preheat the oven to 350°F (180°C) and grease a 12-hole muffin tray or 2 smaller cupcake trays.

Whisk the flour, baking powder, and spices in a bowl and stir in the parsley.

Whisk the eggs, milk, and melted fat in a separate bowl or measuring cup, and pour into the dry ingredients along with the cooled chorizo and chard mixture, and the feta. Using a large spoon, mix only until just combined; do not overmix. Spoon into the greased muffin pans.

Bake in the oven for 25 minutes until golden and a skewer inserted in the center comes out clean (allowing for patches of melted feta). Let cool in the trays for a couple of minutes before turning out onto wire racks to cool completely.

7 oz (200g) traditionally made cooking chorizo (the soft kind), casings removed and broken into small pieces

1 medium onion, finely chopped

10½oz (300g) rainbow or Swiss chard, stalks chopped into small dice, leaves shredded into bite-size pieces

Generous 2 cups (300g) wholewheat spelt flour

1 Tbsp baking powder

1½ tsp smoked paprika

½ tsp cayenne pepper (omit if using spicy chorizo or cooking for children)

1 cup (25g/small bunch) parsley, leaves only, finely chopped

3 medium eggs (about 200g total)

⅝ cup (150ml) whole milk, or milk substitute

2 Tbsp butter, coconut oil, or ghee, melted, plus extra for greasing

Scant 1⅔ cups (200g) feta cheese, crumbled

Sea salt

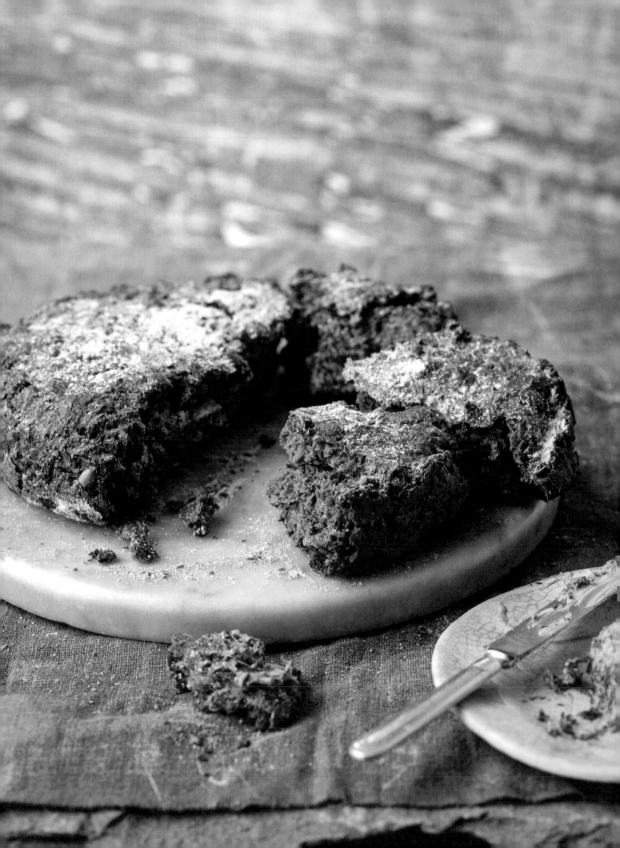

Collard greens and pumpkin seed rye "sourdough"

This is not strictly sourdough, but the long rising time gives the bread a complex, delicious sourdough taste and makes it a lot easier to digest. It seems cumbersome to make, as there are a few steps, but the effort is well worth it, especially if you crave a proper bread but don't have a sourdough starter. You could always double the recipe and make two loaves, slicing and freezing one for later use. Serve with an omelet or a selection of cheeses and chutneys. MAKES 1 SMALL PILLOW LOAF

Steam or sauté the greens in a little water until wilted. Drain and let cool, then very finely chop or process in a food processor.

In a large bowl, combine the greens, flour, yeast, salt, and pumpkin and caraway seeds. Add the water and stir until blended. The dough will be shaggy and sticky. Cover the bowl with plastic wrap and let the dough rest for at least 12 hours, but preferably about 18 to 20 hours, at warm room temperature. The dough is ready when it feels spongy when pressed with a finger. If you break it open slightly, you will see the threads that have developed.

Scrape the dough out onto a lightly floured counter. Sprinkle it with a little more flour and fold it over on itself a couple of times. You should not have to get your hands dirty to do this. Cover loosely with the plastic wrap and let rest for 15 minutes.

Using just enough flour to keep the dough from sticking to the counter or to your fingers, gently shape the dough into a ball. Again, you should use enough flour not to get your hands dirty.

Place a large piece of plastic wrap or a cotton dishtowel on a tray and generously dust with flour. Place the dough on it seam side down, dust with more flour, and cover with a second piece of plastic wrap or towel. Let rise again, 3 to 4 hours, in a warm place. The dough should more than double in size and the surface should crack.

At least 30 minutes before you are ready to bake the bread, preheat the oven to 450°F (230°C). Choose a lidded, heavy-bottom (cast iron, enamel, Pyrex, or ceramic) pot or dish that will neatly fit the dough (about 8in/20cm) and put the pot (without the lid) in the oven as it heats.

When the dough is ready, carefully remove the hot pot from the oven. Slide your hand under the plastic wrap under the dough and carefully turn the dough over into the pot. Be careful not to let dough fold over onto itself. It may look a little messy, but give the pot a shake to evenly distribute the dough.

Cover with the lid and bake for 30 minutes, then lower the oven temperature to 350°F (180°C) and bake for another 70 minutes, until beautifully brown, with a lovely crust. Turn out onto a wire rack and cool completely before cutting. It freezes well in slices and can be toasted from frozen.

10½oz (300g) collard greens, thick core and stalks removed, roughly chopped

4 cups (450g) rye flour, plus extra for dusting

¼ tsp active dry yeast

1¼ tsp fine sea salt

¾ cup (100g) pumpkin seeds

2 tsp caraway seeds (optional)

1⅔ cups (400ml) tepid water

Broccoli and beet greens pie

Ras-el-hanout is a classic spice mixture used in Moroccan cuisine. The name means "top of the shop," which reflects its expensive ingredients, and good mixtures will contain more than 20 different spices, and up to 100. It is available from most major grocery stores and ethnic grocers, but if you feel up to it, you can easily make it yourself (see page 155). Use chard if you can't find beet greens. If you are short of time, you could replace the roasted tomatoes with sliced fresh tomatoes, placed in a single layer on top of the other veg. SERVES 4 (OR 6 AS AN APPETIZER)

For the dough, put the flour, salt, turmeric, and butter in a food processor and pulse until the mixture resembles wet sand. Alternatively, you can do this by hand, by rubbing the butter into the dough with your fingertips. Pulse or stir in the cold water a little at a time until the dough comes together into a ball. Tip the dough onto a counter and knead briefly until smooth; it shouldn't be sticky or crumbly.

Shape the dough into a flat disk and roll it out to about ⅛in (3mm) between two sheets of baking parchment (the dough sheet can be either round or square-ish). Refrigerate until firm.

For the filling, steam the green beans and broccoli separately until just tender; be careful not to overcook. Refresh under cold running water and set aside.

Sauté the beet stalks in the butter, ghee, or coconut oil with a pinch of salt until tender, 5 to 15 minutes, depending on thickness. Add a splash of water to speed along the process if you like. Add the leaves to the pan and cook until wilted, then tip the contents of the pan into a food processor and let cool completely.

Remove the firm dough from the refrigerator and allow to come to room temperature. Preheat the oven to 350°F (180°C).

Add the sour cream, ras-el-hanout, and a little salt to the cooled greens and process together.

Place the dough, still on the baking parchment, on a large baking sheet. Put the green beans in a double layer over the center of the dough, leaving a 2- to 3-in (5- to 8-cm) empty border all round. Drizzle the beans with olive oil and balsamic vinegar, and sprinkle with a little salt.

Spread half the Slow-Roasted Cherry Tomatoes on top of the beans, then spoon the beet greens on top evenly, and top with the rest of the tomatoes. Arrange the broccoli on top and finish with a generous drizzle of oil and sprinkle of salt. Fold the edges of the dough up and over the filling on all sides, pinching together in places to ensure the dough doesn't slide down; the filling should still be visible in the center.

If you are using the egg wash, dip a brush in the beaten egg and lightly brush the pastry with it. Bake for 35 minutes or until the pastry is golden and crunchy. Cool slightly before serving.

FOR THE PIE DOUGH

1⅔ cups (225g) wholewheat flour

Pinch of sea salt

Generous ½ tsp ground turmeric

7 Tbsp cold, unsalted butter, diced

3 to 4 Tbsp ice-cold water

FOR THE FILLING

3½oz (100g/a good handful) of fine green beans, trimmed

5¼oz (150g) tenderstem broccoli (or regular broccoli, cut into smaller pieces)

7oz (200g) tender beet greens, stalks finely chopped, leaves cut into bite-size pieces

A little butter, ghee, or coconut oil

¾ cup (180ml) sour cream

1½ tsp ras-el-hanout (see page 155 to make your own)

Extra-virgin olive oil

Aged balsamic vinegar

7oz (200g) Slow-Roasted Cherry Tomatoes (page 154)

1 egg, lightly beaten, to glaze (optional)

Sea salt

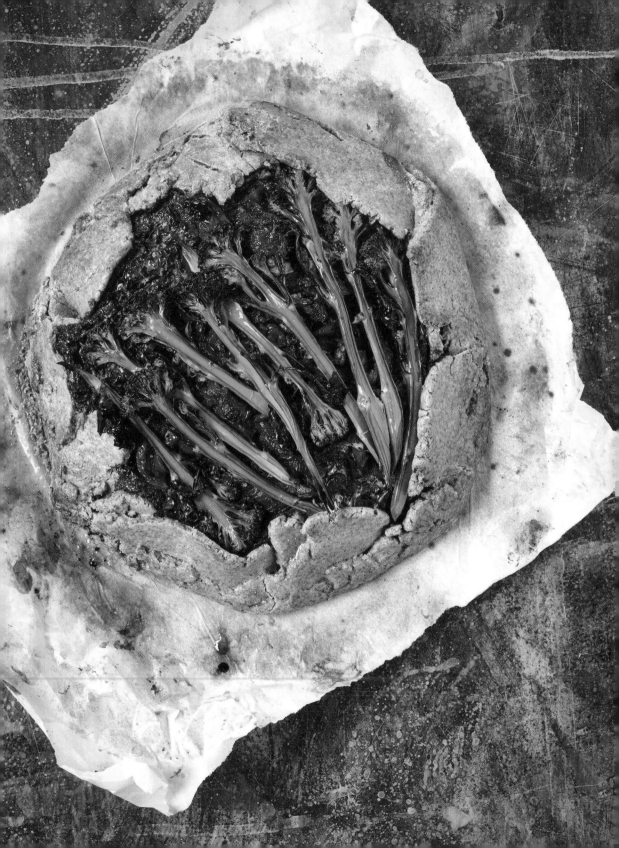

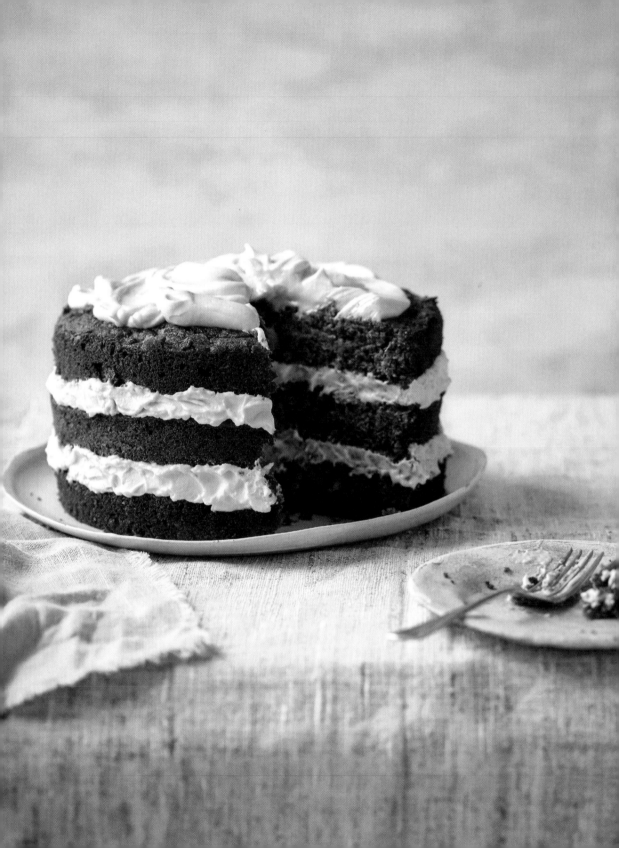

Apple and green cabbage cake

This makes a rather impressive three-tier cake that is deliciously moist, has telltale green flecks, and a wonderful flavor. The frosting is also good with a bit of heavy cream whisked into the cream cheese instead of butter. Buy a few pots of organic pureed apple in the baby section of your grocery store, or make your own by cooking down some apples and blitzing into a puree, then freeze what you don't need in ice-cube trays. Try to find organic dried apple, as it is chewier than nonorganic. SERVES 8 TO 10

Preheat the oven to 350°F (180°C). Grease three 8-in (20-cm) cake pans and line the bottoms with wax paper.

For the cake, whisk together the flour, almond flour, sugar, baking soda, and salt in a bowl. In a separate bowl, whisk together the vanilla seeds, applesauce, eggs, and oil.

Pour the wet ingredients into the dry and whisk until just combined. Stir in the cabbage, grated apple, and dried apple. Pour the batter into the prepared pans and bake for 45 minutes or until springy to the touch and the cake pulls away from the sides of the pan.

Let cool in the pans for about 10 minutes before turning out and cooling completely on a wire rack.

For the frosting, cream the butter with an electric whisk until light and fluffy. Add cream cheese and beat until smooth and well combined, then stir in the maple syrup. Chill in the refrigerator to set slightly before using to sandwich the cake layers and spread over the finished cake.

FOR THE CAKE

2¾ cups (380g) wholewheat spelt flour

½ cup (50g) almond flour or ground almonds

1½ cups packed (280g) dark brown sugar

1 Tbsp baking soda

1 tsp sea salt

1 vanilla bean, split lengthwise and seeds scraped out

1 cup (250ml) applesauce or puree (see Introduction above)

4 large or 5 medium eggs

1½ cups (375ml) liquid coconut oil (about 10½oz/300g solid), macadamia nut oil, or cooking oil of your choice

5 cups (300g) very finely shredded green (sweet) cabbage, chopped up a few times

2 large cooking apples (about 1lb/450g), peeled, cored, and finely grated

¾ cup (70g) chopped dried apple

FOR THE FROSTING

Generous ¾ cup (200g) unsalted butter, at room temperature

1¾ cups (400g) cream cheese, at room temperature

⅓ cup (90ml) maple syrup

Choc-mint ice-cream sandwiches

Perfect for hassle-free entertaining, the ice-cream mixture is made a day in advance, leaving only the churning and assembly for the day. The cookies can be made a day ahead, too. The ice cream needs a good 4 to 6 hours in the freezer after it has been churned, so take this into account when you plan your to-do list. It will seem like a lot of mint to use, but it's correct, and gives an amazing depth of flavor! The ice cream is also fantastic on its own. MAKES 8

For the ice cream, put the chopped mint in a saucepan with the cream and milk and heat until the milk steams—just before it starts to boil. Immediately remove from the heat and let cool for 15 minutes. Repeat this step once (or, if you have time, twice) more. Strain the mixture, using the back of a large spoon to press every last drop of minty-ness out of the leaves, then discard them.

Whisk together the eggs and sugar. Add the mint and cream mixture in a thin, steady stream, whisking continuously. Return the mixture to the pan and cook over low heat, stirring constantly, until it has thickened slightly and coats the back of a wooden spoon. Do not allow to boil or overheat, as the eggs will scramble.

As soon as the custard has thickened, remove from the heat and set the pan in a bowl of cold water (add ice if you have it) to cool. Refrigerate the mixture overnight, then add the chocolate chips and churn in an ice-cream machine according to the manufacturer's directions. Alternatively, you could freeze it in a large, flat container, removing it every hour to break up the ice crystals with a stick blender or electric whisk. Ideally freeze the ice cream in a flat container that will yield a frozen slab ¾ to 1¼in (2 to 3cm) thick, for 4 to 6 hours, or until firm.

For the cookies, preheat the oven to 350°F (180°C) and line a large baking sheet with baking parchment.

In a bowl, whisk together the flour, baking powder, salt, and cocoa powder; set aside. Using an electric mixer, cream the butter and sugar together until light and fluffy. Add the egg and mix until blended. Add the dry ingredients and mix until just combined.

Use a tablespoon to drop 16 even-size amounts of dough onto the prepared baking sheet, leaving some space between each. Use the back of the spoon to flatten each cookie, dipping the spoon in a glass of water in between. Bake for 10 minutes, or until set around the edges but still soft in the center; take care not to overbake. Remove from the oven and leave on the baking tray for a few minutes before transferring to a wire rack to cool.

To assemble, portion out balls of ice cream with an ice-cream scoop, or cut out circles with a cookie cutter, place on the underside of a cookie, and top with another cookie. Eat immediately or freeze until ready to eat.

FOR THE ICE CREAM
6⅔ cups (200g) mint leaves, finely chopped

1½ cups (375ml) heavy cream

1½ cups (375ml) whole milk or milk substitute

2 large eggs

¾ cup (150g) unrefined superfine sugar, or slightly less if you prefer it less sweet

½ cup (90g) dark chocolate chips or buttons

FOR THE COOKIES
¾ cup plus 2 Tbsp (125g) wholewheat spelt flour

½ tsp baking powder

Pinch of sea salt

⅓ cup (35g) unsweetened cocoa, sifted

⅓ cup (75g) unsalted butter, at room temperature

½ cup (100g) dark brown sugar

1 large egg

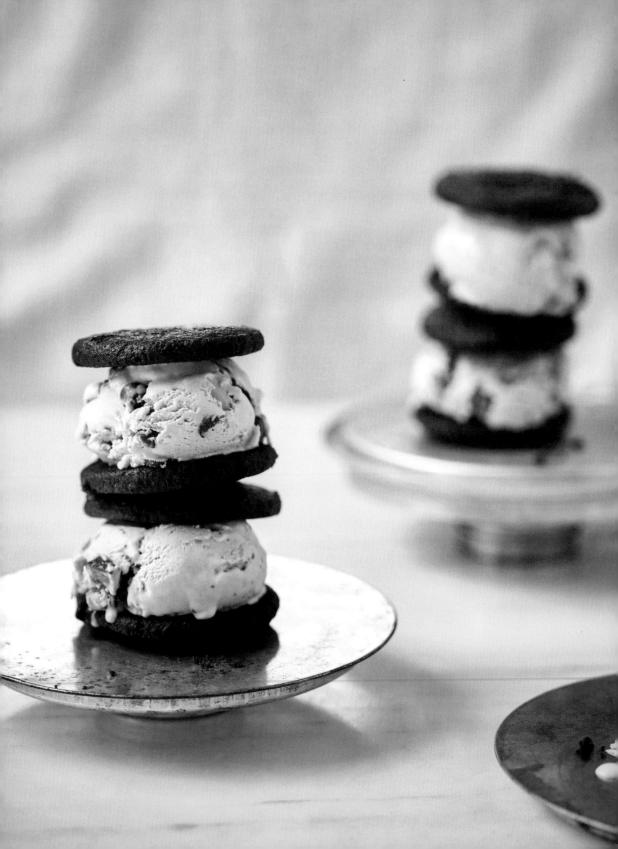

Sweet potato and nettle coconut loaf

If, like me, you often tear your hair out trying to find the perfect savory afternoon (or after-school) snack, this one is for you. A snack should be regarded as a mini-meal—a good balance of protein, healthy fats, and complex carbohydrates. And, of course, some greens! Don't let the number of eggs put you off as they are partly the reason this is such a nutritious snack or side dish. You can easily substitute the wilted nettle with wilted spinach, as long as you squeeze out the liquid. You could also add a little chili, cayenne powder, or fresh herbs, such as chives, to the batter if you like. Coconut flour is available in healthfood stores and major grocery stores. MAKES ABOUT 10 SLICES

Preheat the oven to 350°F (180°C) and line a small loaf pan with baking parchment.

Bring a pan of water to a boil. Protecting your hands, transfer the nettle tips to the boiling water and blanch very briefly until wilted. Drain and cool (keep the liquid to drink as a herbal infusion, or to feed your plants) then squeeze out all the liquid; you should end up with about 1¾ to 2oz (50 to 55g). Chop very finely.

Beat the eggs with the melted butter or oil, using electric beaters or in a stand mixer, until light and airy. Mix in the chopped nettles, sweet potato, coconut flour, flax, sunflower and nigella seeds, spices and baking powder, with a very larch pinch of salt, and some black pepper. Mix until combined.

Transfer the batter to the prepared loaf pan and top with extra sunflower and nigella seeds. Let stand for 10 minutes before baking in the oven for 45 to 55 minutes, or until golden-brown on top and a skewer inserted in the center comes out clean, or with a few dry crumbs attached.

Let cool in the pan for a few minutes before turning out onto a wire rack to cool completely. Slice when cold, butter generously and serve with a spicy bean dip.

2½ oz (70g) nettle tips

8 large or 9 medium eggs, at room temperature

½ cup (125ml) melted butter, ghee, or coconut oil

1 cup (100g) coarsely grated sweet potato (no need to peel)

¾ cup (70g) coconut flour

Scant ½ cup (25g) ground flaxseed or flax meal

¼ cup (35g) sunflower seeds, plus a few extra for the top

1 Tbsp nigella (black onion) seeds, plus a few extra for the top

¼ tsp ground allspice

½ tsp ground ginger

1 tsp ground turmeric (or 1 heaping tsp freshly grated)

½ tsp baking powder

Sea salt and freshly ground black pepper

Honey and thyme buckwheat cookies

These cookies are very different and, as far as treats go, quite nutritious. Both thyme and honey are highly prized for their antibacterial properties, and manuka honey in particular is used by many to treat burns and cuts. Buckwheat, a fruit seed related to rhubarb and sorrel, is not a true cereal and therefore suitable for people with grain and gluten intolerances. It has numerous health benefits and a delicious, distinct taste. MAKES 20 TO 24

Preheat the oven to 320°F (160°C) and line a large baking sheet with baking parchment.

Spread the nuts out on the baking sheet and roast for 10 to 15 minutes, until golden. Remove from the oven and let cool.

Meanwhile, beat the butter and sugar together for a couple of minutes, until creamy and lighter than when you started. Add the thyme and honey and beat for another few seconds to combine, before mixing in the egg yolk.

Put the cooled nuts, flour, and salt in a food processor and blitz until the mixture resembles very coarse sand, making sure you don't grind the nuts too finely. Carefully fold the flour mixture into butter mixture.

Divide the dough (which will be quite sticky and soft) in half and roll each half out between two large sheets of baking parchment to about a ¼in (5mm) thickness. Refrigerate the sheets of dough for about 30 minutes, or until completely firm.

Remove one sheet of dough, cut it into cookie-size rectangles and carefully transfer each cookie to the lined baking sheet, using a spatula. Repeat with the second sheet of dough, returning the dough to the refrigerator to firm up as soon as it gets too sticky to work with.

Bake for about 15 minutes, or until very golden, rotating the sheet once during baking. Remove from the oven and transfer to a wire rack to cool completely.

⅝ cup (75g) shelled, unroasted cashews

⅓ cup (75g) butter, softened

2½ Tbsp unrefined brown cane sugar

1 scant Tbsp very finely chopped thyme leaves

2 Tbsp honey (ideally thyme honey)

1 egg yolk

¾ cup (100g) buckwheat flour

Pinch of sea salt

Zucchini and rosemary chocolate brownies

I won't pretend that these are überhealthy, but the zucchini adds a delicious fluffiness, and if you resist having the whole lot in one go, they are a wonderful treat. I use dark chocolate, but if your audience prefers the sweeter taste of milk chocolate, use that instead. MAKES 16 MEDIUM SQUARES

Preheat the oven to 350°F (180°C). Grease a square cake or brownie pan, about 8in (20cm), and line with baking parchment.

Cut the zucchini in half lengthwise and scrape out the seeds with a spoon. Grate the flesh and set aside in a strainer over a bowl to get rid of excess moisture. You need 200g of grated zucchini.

Put the chocolate into a heatproof bowl, sit over a pan of simmering water, making sure the bottom of the bowl is not touching the water, and let melt, stirring occasionally. Alternatively, you can melt it in a microwave. Set aside to cool.

In a large mixing bowl, whisk together the flour, salt, baking powder, cocoa, and rosemary.

In a separate bowl, cream together the butter and sugar (it's a good idea to check dark brown sugar for any lumps and crush them between thumb and index finger before creaming). Add the eggs one at a time, beating briefly between each addition.

Briefly beat the milk into the egg mixture, before folding in the dry ingredients, chocolate buttons, and walnuts, using a large metal spoon.

Stir in the cooled melted chocolate and then the grated zucchini. Do not overmix; stir just enough to combine. Scrape the batter into the prepared pan and press it into the corners, smoothing the top.

Bake in the oven for 30 to 40 minutes (depending on the size of your pan), until a skewer inserted into the center comes out clean or with a few dry crumbs attached (allowing for patches of melted chocolate).

Let cool in the pan for a few minutes before turning out onto a rack wire to cool completely. Cut into squares and keep in an airtight container for up to 5 days.

2 to 3 medium zucchini

½ cup plus 1 Tbsp (125g) butter, softened, plus extra to grease

4oz (120g) dark (70%) chocolate, broken into pieces

1 cup plus 2 Tbsp (160g) wholewheat spelt flour (or half wholewheat and half white)

Pinch of sea salt

2 tsp baking powder

About 3 Tbsp unsweetened cocoa, sifted

1½ tsp very finely chopped rosemary

⅔ cup (125g) light or dark brown sugar

2 medium eggs

⅝ cup (155 ml) milk of your choice (I use almond)

½ cup (70g) milk chocolate buttons, chips, or roughly chopped squares

Generous ¾ cup (80g) shelled, unroasted walnuts, finely chopped

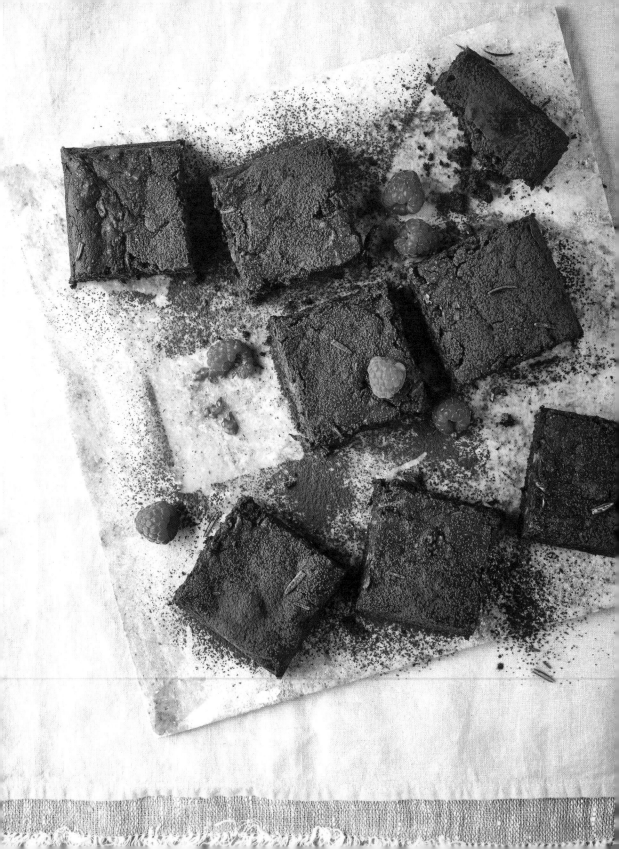

Raw lemon and lime curd tartlets

This is my version of a popular dessert in the raw food world. I love the refreshing, not-too-sweet taste and the fact that it is supremely satisfying. If you've never sprouted anything before, buckwheat chips are the perfect introduction to the world of these enzyme-rich and nutrient-dense foods. Raw buckwheat is available from most healthfood stores, sprouts easily, and the chips are a slightly nuttier version of rice crispies, which can be sprinkled on oatmeal or mixed into granola recipes. You can soak, sprout, and dry the buckwheat well in advance, and keep it in an airtight jar. MAKES 6 TARTLETS

Blitz all the ingredients for the crust in a food processor until the mixture resembles coarse, wet sand. Scrape out and press into 6 mini tart pans, 4in (10cm) diameter. Refrigerate while you make the filling.

In a powerful blender, blend all the ingredients for the filling until very smooth. If using a regular blender, the result will not be quite as smooth, so you may want to strain the mixture through a strainer. Taste, and if it is too tart, add another Tbsp or two of honey, bearing in mind that the crust is sweet and offsets the filling beautifully.

Spoon the filling into the tart shells and refrigerate for at least 4 hours. Carefully unmold each tart and serve with fresh blueberries and some fresh lime or lemon zest. They keep well in their pans in the refrigerator for a day or two.

NOTE:
To sprout raw, unroasted buckwheat (not kasha), soak 2 cups of buckwheat groats in three times their volume of fresh water for 12 to 18 hours, changing the water (it will go slimy) once during this time. Then drain, rinse off any sliminess, and leave for a day or two in a sprouting jar, mesh bag, or strainer, loosely covered with a piece of paper towel or cloth, rinsing well and giving a stir twice a day. Once most of the grains have started sprouting (you will see a tiny little tail forming), spread them all out on a tray or baking sheet and dry in a dehydrator or at a very low temperature (about 149°F/65°C) in the oven until crisp, usually for 12 to 24 hours. The low temperature is essential to preserve the enzymes in the sprouts, but if you are pressed for time, you could increase the temperature and reduce the baking time.

FOR THE CRUST
½ cup (80g) sprouted, dried buckwheat (see Note below)

1½ Tbsp melted coconut oil

1 cup (125g) shelled, unroasted cashews, soaked for a few hours and drained

Grated zest of 1 lemon, plus extra to serve

¾ cup (55g) dry unsweetened coconut

Pinch of sea salt

5 large soft Medjool dates, pitted and chopped

FOR THE FILLING
Scant 1 cup (120g) shelled, unroasted macadamia or pecan nuts, soaked for a few hours then drained

¾ cup (180ml) mixture of lemon and lime juice (about 2 large lemons and 3 limes)

2 large avocados (260 to 280g each), peeled and pitted

¼ cup (60ml) honey

Pinch of sea salt

1 tsp good-quality lemon extract or a few drops of lemon oil

2 Tbsp liquid coconut oil

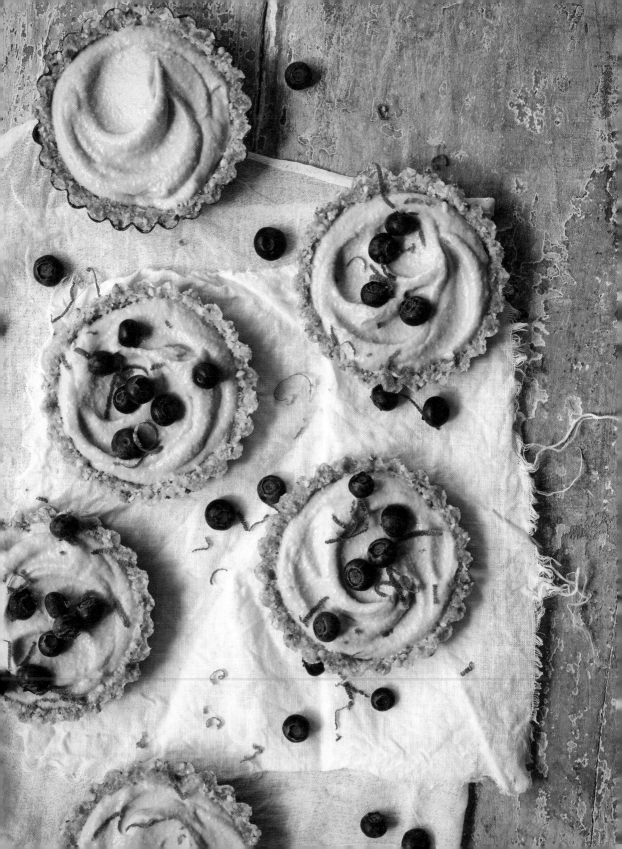

Basic recipes

Cooking legumes

My rough rule of thumb for beans in general is that they will yield 2½ to 3 times the volume (give or take a bit) and twice the weight (give or take a bit) after an overnight soak and cooking. Once rehydrated, beans cook in 15 minutes to 1½ hours, depending on the type of bean. There is much differing opinion on whether to add salt during cooking or after, as some cooks believe it prevents legumes from becoming tender. In my experience this has never happened, and I find a bland bean quite a challenge to eat, so I am in the camp of adding a pinch of salt to the cooking liquid.

Scant 1 to 1 cup (150 to 200g) dried beans or lentils

½ tsp baking soda

1 bay leaf

1 small onion, peeled and quartered

1 to 2 garlic cloves, bruised and peeled

Pinch of sea salt

5 black peppercorns (optional)

Small strip (about 1¼- by 2-in/3- by 5-cm) of kombu/kelp (optional)

Soak the beans or lentils in four times the volume of fresh, room-temperature water and the baking soda for at least 12 hours, but up to 36 hours.

Change the soaking water once a day if you soak for longer than a 24-hour period.

When ready to cook, rinse the beans under cold running water, then place in a saucepan with plenty of fresh water, the bay leaf, onion, garlic, salt, peppercorns, and kombu/kelp, if using.

Bring the water to a boil, then turn down the heat and simmer with the lid on until the beans are tender. If you plan to use the cooking liquid later, you can boil the beans with the lid ajar, or uncovered, for some or all of the cooking time; this will help the liquid reduce and become flavorful.

Cooking time varies according to the type of bean and soaking time (see below), but it will take anything between 15 minutes to 1½ hours. Taste more than one bean to be sure they are tender, as they can cook at unequal rates.

If you do not need the cooking liquid, drain the beans and use them as stated in your recipe.

NOTE:
If you would like to sprout soaked beans or chickpeas before cooking, rinse them and leave them in a strainer, sprouting jar(s), or net for another day or two, or until tiny tails start growing from one end. At this point they are ready to cook.

Cooking time in minutes	Dried legume (1 cup's worth) (after soaking)
10 to 15	black (or Beluga) lentils, Puy lentils, red lentils, split peas
15 to 20	green lentils, brown lentils
30 to 45	aduki beans, whole dried peas
45 to 60	black-eye peas, black beans, fava beans, haricot beans, pinto beans, mung beans, and kidney beans
60 to 90	chickpeas, lima beans, cannellini beans

Rich tomato sauce

This is one of the most versatile staples in my refrigerator, and I usually make a big batch and freeze it in smaller portions. It's great on its own as a pizza or pasta sauce, or as a base for a myriad other sauces and soups. MAKES ABOUT 2 CUPS (500 ML)

2¼lb (1kg) medium to large vine tomatoes (about 9 to 11), halved and fibrous stalks removed

1 whole garlic bulb, skin on, cut in half horizontally

2 large red onions (10½ to 12¼oz/300 to 350g), peeled and quartered

Olive oil

Aged balsamic vinegar

Pinch of cayenne pepper (optional)

Honey (optional)

Sea salt and freshly ground black pepper

Preheat the oven to 300°F (150°C).

Toss the tomatoes and onions in some olive oil and balsamic vinegar, season with salt and pepper, and arrange in a baking sheet, cut sides up. Roast for 2 to 2½ hours.

Rub some olive oil on the cut sides of the garlic, then wrap in foil and add to the oven to roast for at least 1 hour, or until the cloves are soft.

Once roasted, scrape the tomatoes and onions into a blender, squeeze out the soft and squidgy garlic cloves, and blend until smooth. Adjust the seasoning and add the cayenne pepper if you prefer it spicy.

If you're using the sauce as a condiment, add honey to taste

Basic tomato sauce

This has less depth of flavor than the Rich Tomato Sauce and makes a great foundation for many tomato-based dishes. You'll need it for the Collard Greens Lasagna (page 94). MAKES ABOUT 3¾ CUPS (900ML)

Butter, or coconut or olive oil, for frying

1 medium onion, diced

Sea salt

2 garlic cloves, finely chopped

2 x 14-oz (400-g) cans chopped tomatoes

2 Tbsp tomato paste or concentrate

Large pinch of unrefined brown sugar

1 Tbsp balsamic vinegar

Heat some butter, or coconut or olive oil in a medium saucepan and gently sweat the onion until soft and translucent.

Add the garlic and fry for another minute or so, before adding the rest of the ingredients.

Simmer for 15 to 25 minutes or until thick and somewhat reduced. If the sauce is too chunky, use a stick blender to blitz for a few seconds.

Slow-roasted cherry tomatoes

Another versatile staple that I keep in my refrigerator. MAKES 14¾ TO 15¾OZ (425 TO 450G)

2¼lb (1kg) cherry or baby plum tomatoes, halved

Extra-virgin olive oil

Aged balsamic vinegar

Sea salt and freshly ground black pepper

Preheat the oven to 300°F (150°C).

Gently toss the tomato halves in some olive oil and vinegar to coat. Add some salt and pepper, then spread onto a large lipped baking sheet, cut side up and in a single layer.

Roast in the oven for 1½ to 2 hours, depending on how moist you want the tomatoes to be.

Let cool before spooning into jars. Cover and store in the refrigerator for a week or two, or you can freeze them.

Roasted garlic

This makes enough for four servings of Green Celeriac Mash (page 75), but it can easily be frozen or stored in the refrigerator covered with a layer of olive oil for a couple of weeks. If you find yourself making this regularly, invest in a little ovenproof lidded dish for roasting the garlic.

1 whole garlic bulb

Olive oil

Sea salt and freshly ground black pepper

Preheat the oven to 320°F (160°C).

Without removing the outer peel of the bulb of garlic, slice through it horizontally. Rub both cut halves with olive oil. Sprinkle with salt and pepper, then place the cut sides together, wrap the whole bulb in foil, and bake in the oven for 40 to 50 minutes or until the garlic is soft and squidgy.

Squeeze the flesh out of each clove and use it as stated in your recipe.

Tarragon mayonnaise

This keeps well in the refrigerator for a week or so and can be enjoyed with almost anything, from boiled eggs and asparagus, to cucumber sandwiches. One of my favorite ways to use mayonnaise is in Mexican street-style corn, where broiled or barbecued corn is slathered in it, then sprinkled with grated cheese, chili powder, and lime juice. MAKES ABOUT 1 CUP (250ML)

1 egg yolk, at room temperature

1 Tbsp lemon juice

1 tsp Dijon mustard

¾ to 1 cup (180 to 250ml) oil (I usually use a mix: walnut, mild-tasting extra virgin olive, and cold-pressed sunflower, or canola)

⅓ cup (10g/a few sprigs) tarragon, leaves only, finely chopped

1 garlic clove, finely chopped

Sea salt

Put the egg yolk, lemon juice, and mustard in a bowl with a rubber bottom or stand the bowl on a wet dishtowel to stop it moving around while you whisk.

Start whisking the ingredients with a small balloon whisk while adding the oil drop by drop until the mixture starts to thicken (or emulsify). This may take a while, so don't lose patience and be tempted to start adding the oil more quickly.

Once it has thickened slightly, you can start adding the oil in a very thin, steady stream, whisking continuously.

Continue adding the oil until you have reached the desired consistency. Your mayonnaise should look thick and unctuous.

Season with salt and stir in the tarragon and garlic.

Ras-el-hanout spice mix

If you are unable to find any of the ingredients already ground, feel free to grind them yourself using a spice grinder or a mortar and pestle.

½ tsp ground star anise or 1 whole star anise (optional)

Seeds from 4 to 5 cardamom pods, finely ground

½ tsp freshly grated nutmeg

½ tsp mustard powder

1 tsp ground turmeric

1 tsp fine sea salt

1 tsp ground ginger

1 tsp freshly ground black pepper

½ tsp ground cinnamon

½ tsp cayenne pepper

¾ tsp ground coriander

¼ tsp ground cloves

1 tsp ground cumin

½ tsp ground allspice

½ tsp ground fennel seeds

1 tsp edible rose buds (optional)

½ tsp edible lavender, flowers only (optional)

If using whole star anise, grind in a spice or coffee grinder until powdered.

Combine all the ingredients, mix well, and store in an airtight container.

Chinese five-spice powder

Five-spice powder is well known and highly valued across China. It usually contains star anise, cassia (or cinnamon), cloves, fennel, and Sichuan pepper in equal parts. Optionally, ginger, galangal, black cardamom, or even licorice may be added. Ideally the spices should be kept whole and then ground just before usage, so do not make large batches.

1 tsp fennel seeds

1 tsp Szechuan peppercorns

1 tsp ground star anise or 2 whole star anise

1 tsp ground cinnamon

1 tsp ground cloves

Heat a small, heavy-bottomed frying pan over medium heat and dry-roast the fennel seeds and Szechuan peppercorns for a couple of minutes, stirring with a wooden spoon or spatula. Set aside to cool.

Once cooled, grind the fennel, Szechuan pepper, and star anise (if using whole) in a spice or coffee grinder, or a high-speed blender, until powdered.

Mix with the rest of the ingredients and store in an airtight container for up to a few months.

Horseradish sauce

The root of the horseradish plant (a member of the mustard family) resembles a parsnip and is used in cooking for its sharp, distinctive taste. Once peeled, it can be grated and mixed with other ingredients to make spicy sauces to accompany fish or roast beef. Do be careful when you work with horseradish, as it is much more potent than freshly chopped onions and can sting your eyes if you get too close.

MAKES ⅔ CUP (160 ML)

2 Tbsp apple cider vinegar

½ tsp honey

1 tsp Dijon mustard (or if you like it really spicy, hot English mustard)

2 to 3 Tbsp finely grated fresh or jarred horseradish root

½ cup (125ml) sour cream

Sea salt

Combine the vinegar, salt, honey, and mustard in a small bowl. Stir in the grated the horseradish and set aside for 10 minutes to let the flavors meld.

Gradually whisk in the sour cream and add salt to taste. Store in an airtight container in the refrigerator for 2 to 3 weeks.

Sticky brown rice

SERVES 2

Scant 1 cup (150g) short-grain brown rice

Generous 1 cup (280ml) water

Large pinch of sea salt

Rinse the rice under cold running water until the water runs clear. Put into a saucepan with the water and salt.

Cover and bring to a boil, then turn the heat down to low and cook gently and undisturbed for 30 minutes, without lifting the lid at all.

After 30 minutes, check all the water has been absorbed by inserting a knife into the center of the pan and gently pushing aside some of the rice, so you can see the bottom of the pan. If there's still water, cover again and continue to cook for a few minutes, checking regularly.

Once all the water has been absorbed, add approximately the same volume of water as there is rice, erring on the side of less. Mix the water into the rice well, then bring back to a simmer and turn down to low.

Cover and cook as before for 10 to 15 minutes, until all the water has been absorbed. Remove from the heat and let the rice steam for another 5 minutes, with the lid on.

Roasted spiced nuts

Used in the Mexican Rice and Black Bean Salad (page 127), this recipe makes much more than you need, but you will be glad for it, as it is the most moreish snack you could ever wish for.

MAKES 3½ CUPS (500G)

3⅓ cups (500g) mixed shelled, unroasted nuts (Brazils, pecans, walnuts, almonds, hazelnuts, cashews)

1 egg white, lightly whisked

½ to 1 Tbsp finely flaked sea salt

2 tsp ground cumin

1 tsp garlic powder

1 heaping tsp ground dried oregano

2 tsp sweet paprika

2 tsp dried chipotle chili powder

Preheat the oven to 320°F (160°C) and line a baking sheet with baking parchment.

Stir the nuts into the egg white to coat, then add the spices and mix well. Spread out in a single layer on the lined baking sheet and bake in the oven for 30 minutes or until crisp and crunchy, giving them a stir halfway through.

Vegan Greek-style "yogurt"

MAKES ABOUT ¾ CUP (200 ML)

3½oz (100g) young coconut meat without the water

¼ cup (35g) shelled, unroasted macadamia nuts, soaked in cold water for 4 hours then drained

1½ Tbsp lemon juice

Pinch of sea salt

1 tsp probiotic powder, or the contents of a probiotic capsule

Blend all the ingredients in a high-speed blender, or with a stick blender, until smooth. Store in an airtight container in the refrigerator for up to 1 week.

Macadamia nut spread

It is hard to imagine something being refreshing and utterly unctuous at the same time, but this dairy-free spread delivers on both those fronts. Serve dollops of it with salads or roasted vegetables, or mix with hummus for a fantastic dip. MAKES ABOUT 1 CUP (250ML)

1 cup (140g) shelled, unroasted macadamia nuts, soaked in cold water for a few hours then drained

1½ Tbsp lemon juice

Pinch of salt

½ Tbsp nutritional yeast flakes (optional)

1 tsp maple syrup

1 Tbsp olive oil

2 to 4 Tbsp water, as needed

In the small bowl of a food processor, or using a stick blender, pulse together all the ingredients until the spread has a relatively smooth consistency, with a few crunchy bits.

Resources

Raw and grass-fed dairy products

organicpastures.com

eatwild.com

Thai young coconuts and raw coconut water

melissas.com

vitacoco.com

Grains, nuts, dried fruit, "superfoods" etc.

vitacost.com

iHerb.com

sunfood.com

Grass-fed meat, and preservative-free sausages and bacon

eatwild.com

grasslandbeef.com

goodearthfarms.com

Index

Acknowledgments

I would like to express my deeply felt gratitude to the many people who have been instrumental in making this book possible.

- My fantastic team of recipe testers spread across the globe: Helen Butterworth, Florence Murray, Ida Marie Rasmussen, Vera Cottrell, Marijke Peters, Marianne Brammer, Anneke and Chris Herselman, Melissa Kuzma, Pascaline Monier, Anna Hopwood, Erika Wagner, Catherine and Gary Hoff, Melissa Slomienski, and Caroline Fowler

- My editor, Céline Hughes, for sharing my enthusiasm when I first expressed the idea, and whose attention to detail and calm presence have been equally valuable in seeing it through

- Nassima Rothacker, whose beautiful images will no doubt inspire readers to make every single recipe in this book

- Nikki Ellis, for her artistic guidance and hard work in creating a breathtaking end result

- Food stylist extraordinaire, Aya Nishimura, who steadily churned out dishes AND made them look beautiful

And finally, a HUGE thank you to the three boys in my life who eat the food I serve them with hearty appetites and (almost always) without complaint. You are the reason I go that extra mile.

Publishing Director: Sarah Lavelle
Creative Director: Helen Lewis
Senior Editor: Céline Hughes
Designer: Nicola Ellis
Photographer: Nassima Rothacker
Food Stylist: Aya Nishimura
Prop Stylist: Polly Webb-Wilson
Production: Vincent Smith, Emily Noto

First published in 2016 by
Quadrille Publishing
Pentagon House
52–54 Southwark Street
London SE1 1UN
www.quadrille.com

Quadrille is an imprint of Hardie Grant
www.hardiegrant.com.au

Text © 2016 Zita Steyn
All photography © 2016 Nassima Rothacker
Design and layout © 2016 Quadrille Publishing

ISBN: 978 184949 916 3
Printed in China

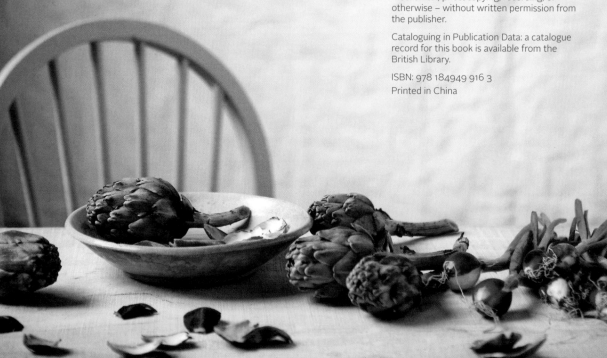